Nutritional Care for Older People

A guide to good practice

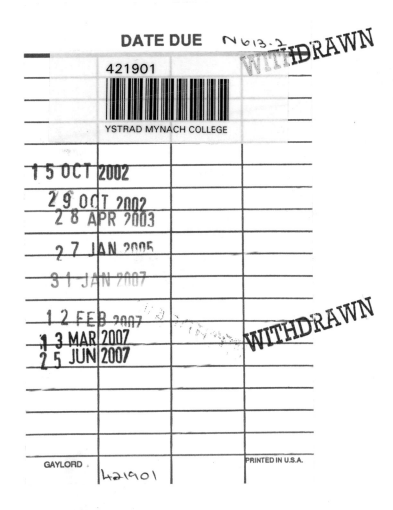

care professional handbook series

Nutritional Care for Older People

A guide to good practice

June Copeman

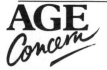

AGE Concern

BOOKS

© 1999 June Copeman

Published by Age Concern England
1268 London Road
London SW16 4ER

First published 1999

Editor Ro Lyon
Production Vinnette Marshall
Design and typesetting GreenGate Publishing Services
Printed in Great Britain by Bell & Bain Ltd, Glasgow

A catalogue record for this book is available from the British Library.

ISBN 0-86242-284-1

While every effort has been made to check the accuracy of material contained in this publication, Age Concern England cannot accept responsibility for the results of any action taken by readers as a result of reading this book. Please note that while the agencies or products mentioned in this book are known to Age Concern, inclusion here does not constitute a recommendation by Age Concern for any particular product, agency, service or publication.

Bulk orders
Age Concern England is pleased to offer customised editions of all its titles to UK companies, institutions or other organisations wishing to make a bulk purchase. For further information, please contact the Publishing Department at the address on this page. Tel: 020 8765 7200. Fax: 020 8765 7211. E-mail: addisom@ace.org.uk

CONTENTS

ABOUT THE AUTHOR

June Copeman BSc, MSc, Med, SRD is Senior Lecturer in Nutrition and Dietetics at Leeds Metropolitan University. She is a State Registered Dietitian who worked in several NHS Trusts and overseas before moving into higher education in 1988.

Her particular interest in the nutrition of older people began in 1985 when she was involved in establishing a dietetic service for older people in Wales. Since then she has contributed to the post-registration education and training of dietitians working with older people across the UK as course leader and as Chair of the Nutrition Advisory Group for Elderly People (NAGE) of the British Dietetic Association (1991-98).

In 1994-95 she was a member of the Caroline Walker Trust Expert Working Party which produced *Eating Well for Older People: Practical and nutritional guidelines for food in residential and nursing homes and for community meals*.

She has spoken at many national and regional voluntary sector events about the nutrition needs of older people and acted as a spokesperson to the media. June has written widely in the care sector journals and is co-author with Dr G Webb of *The Nutrition of Older Adults* (1996).

ACKNOWLEDGEMENTS

I would like to thank the members of the Nutrition Advisory Group for Elderly People (NAGE) of the British Dietetic Association for their support, encouragement and constructive comments during the development of this book. I am particularly indebted to Rev P Eaton SRD for her thoughts and our discussions on the religious and cultural roles of food (Chapter 2).

Thanks also go to Dr Geof Webb. Working with Dr Webb in our earlier joint publication, *The Nutrition of Older Adults*, helped me to confirm the key issues in relation to nutrition and older people and this book therefore reflects our joint work. The chapter on nutritional assessment (Chapter 6) most explicitly draws on this work.

Finally I would like to express my appreciation to the people in the many voluntary sector groups who have helped me to refine my ideas and to the older people who have offered suggestions and told me when the information was unrealistic.

June Copeman

INTRODUCTION

This book aims to provide useful information about nutrition issues that are relevant and important to older people. It seeks to make carers more aware of the importance of food, in its broadest sense, to the well-being of their older clients. It is intended to be particularly of use to the proprietors, managers and staff of residential homes, day centres, meals on wheels services and community catering services for older people. It aims to increase your knowledge, enable you to identify nutrition issues and suggest when and how to intervene to encourage older people to eat and drink. The practical suggestions are intended to help you offer more appropriate nutritional care.

Reading this book will enable you to:

- examine your own attitudes to, and assumptions about, food and food selection and consider how these could affect your working practices;
- understand why some older people are reluctant to eat and drink;
- identify nutrition issues that are important to older people;
- recognise common nutritional problems affecting older people;
- explain how an adequate nutritional intake can improve the quality of life for many people with chronic illness;
- offer practical assistance to enable older people to eat and drink; *and*
- consider what institutional changes are needed to ensure that older people receive an adequate food intake.

The book is divided into eight chapters:

Chapter 1 identifies the changes involved in the normal ageing process that have an impact in relation to the nutrition of older people.

Chapter 2 examines the importance of food and its various roles. Factors affecting food intake and eating patterns are considered, including the importance of past experience, culture and religious belief.

Chapter 3 presents the current nutritional guidelines and recommendations for nutritional requirements. The nutritional adequacy of the diets of older people is discussed. Information is also provided about the Caroline Walker Trust guidelines for the nutritional content of community and residential meals.

Chapter 4 examines group catering issues. It considers strategies to improve nutritional status at an institutional level, including the importance of adequate menu planning and the service and presentation of meals.

Chapter 5 looks at some nutrition issues that are of importance for healthier older people – constipation, anaemia, obesity, hyperlipidaemia and diabetes – conditions which can occur at any age but are more common among older people. The condition and general guidelines on dietary treatment are described in each case.

Chapter 6 describes the techniques used to assess the nutritional status of an individual. The importance of nutritional screening to identify people at risk of malnutrition in the community and on admission to residential care or hospital is highlighted.

Chapter 7 addresses the issue of stimulating a small appetite and offers practical suggestions about using food supplements. Techniques to encourage fluid intake, including a food and fluid chart, are described. Advice is given on how to assist an individual who has difficulty swallowing and also on what to do when someone cannot eat or drink orally.

Chapter 8 examines the particular needs of older people with dementia.

Eleven case studies are included in the text. If possible try to discuss your answers to the questions with other people. The answer section at the end of the book offers a list of possible issues that you would have been expected to consider but you may well have thought of other suggestions to help solve each problem.

The book concludes with a glossary to explain technical terms. Also included are suggestions for further reading and useful addresses, a list of the tables and an index to help you find your way around the book.

1 How Ageing Impacts on Nutrition

This chapter sets the scene by briefly examining the implications of increased life expectancy and the significance of the normal ageing process in relation to the nutrition of older people.

An ageing population

Ageing is a continuous process and deciding when someone is old is arbitrary. The World Health Organisation (WHO) uses chronological age in the following classification: 60-74 elderly; 75-89 old; 90+ very old. In the UK it is customary to consider 65 years, the retirement age for men, as the start of old age. The older population is, of course, diverse, covering over thirty years and in this book we use the term 'older people' except when quoting from other publications.

The number of older people is increasing worldwide. In the UK there are over 10 million pensioners, representing about 18 per cent of the population. Throughout Europe older people represent about 20 per cent of the total population, but this will increase to 25 per cent by 2020. This increase in the proportion of older people in the population is due to fewer children being born and more people reaching old age.

Life expectancy is one measure of the health of populations. In 1901 life expectancy in the UK was 49 years for men and 45 years for women. By 1995 this had risen to 74.3 years for men and 79.5 years for women (World Health Organisation 1998). This dramatic rise in life expectancy has occurred because less people have died in infancy and childhood from infectious diseases.

Unfortunately this rise in life expectancy cannot always be disability and disease free. On average a woman can expect to live 16 years of her life with some form of disability and a man about 14 years. One of the challenges of the twenty-first century will be to reduce the number of years people live with a disability in later life; to improve the quality of life as we age.

Older people aged 65–75 are generally fit and active members of the community and have a health profile similar to younger middle-aged people. As people become older the likelihood of developing a chronic illness and subsequent disability increases. Therefore the need for support from others in the community increases; many people over 85 years receive some formal or informal support.

The proportion of people aged over 80 is the fastest growing section of the British population. In 1951 three hundred people were aged 100 years; by 2031 this will be 34,000 (*British Medical Journal* editorial 1997). This increase in the number of people in the oldest age group means that the need for home support in the community and for residential and nursing home care will increase.

Most older people prefer to live in their own homes for as long as possible; therefore the need for domiciliary services including community meals will also grow. The services provided must be appropriate and meet the needs of the client. In nutrition terms this means that the client has the opportunity to consume a wide variety of food in sufficient quantity to meet their nutritional requirements.

In recent years there has been an increase in the number of older people living in residential and nursing homes. Although the absolute number has increased, the percentage of the age group is still only about 5 per cent. These older people are dependent on others for their food and other needs; therefore the provision of appropriate food is essential to their survival and sense of well-being.

Normal changes in the ageing process

Ageing is a normal process involving a range of physiological and biochemical changes. These changes may influence the presentation of a disease, the response to treatment and likelihood of ensuing complications. Various organs and systems in the body degenerate at different rates – for example circulation, respiration and skin – but all are affected.

Four issues that are particularly important to the general nutrition of older people are: physical fitness and strength; skeletal changes; fluid balance and renal (kidney) function; and the impact of ageing on the immune system (Webb and Copeman 1996). Changes in the gut and sensory organs are also significant as they directly influence the inclination and ability of an individual to eat.

Physical fitness and strength

Physical activity and fitness are important throughout life. Regular exercise, preferably aerobic, can benefit all ages. It increases muscle strength and the ability of the circulatory and respiratory systems to deliver oxygen to all parts of the body. It also improves flexibility, which can be important in encouraging mobility. Typical aerobic exercise, such as brisk walking and energetic housework, increase the heart rate and should be incorporated into everyday activities. Weight bearing exercises, where the body carries its own weight, such as walking, also help to maintain the strength of the bones and are doubly valuable. Being more active and undertaking exercise has been shown to be of benefit to older people. Even chair-bound individuals should be encouraged to exercise their upper body with a programme including bicep curls and other arm movements. Where possible leg and feet exercises (such as rotating the ankle) should be included as part of activities at your residential home or day centre.

Skeletal changes

A decline in body height as we age is caused by vertebral (backbone) disc degeneration and compression. The bone density is reduced because of increased reabsorption of calcium which means that the cortex (outer part) of the bones becomes weak and more liable to fracture. Fractures are very common in older women due to osteoporosis. After the menopause the rate of reabsorption of calcium increases and becomes greater than the amount being laid down and so the bone becomes weaker and more brittle. Decalcification starts earlier and is affected by a diet which is low in calcium and by limited weight bearing exercise and other factors. Experts disagree as to whether the body can respond to a therapeutic increase in calcium. There is, however, general agreement that older people should eat a diet rich in calcium from such sources as milk and undertake regular physical activities to slow down the decalcification process.

Fluid balance and renal function

The composition of the whole body changes during ageing. There is decline in the amount of lean body tissue, an increase in body fat and a decrease in the percentage of body water. This means that older people can have impaired temperature regulation, starting to shiver later in response to cold. They are thus more vulnerable to hypothermia.

The reduced renal (kidney) function (meaning that urine cannot be as concentrated) and the decline in the thirst mechanism puts an older person at greater risk of dehydration. Older people thus need to drink plenty of fluids even if they do not feel thirsty.

Changes in the immune system

The immune system has three main functions in helping the body fight infections – recognising abnormal growth in the body's own cells; destroying foreign materials; and acting in the recycling of worn out body cells.

The high incidence of infection in the young child and very old person suggests that at both ends of the lifespan the immune system is compromised. Older people, particularly the more vulnerable, are more susceptible to infection and take longer to recover compared to younger healthy people.

When someone is malnourished their immune system is depressed, ie they are more susceptible to a severe infection. The immune system is also suppressed by some drugs, by disease and by radiotherapy. In parallel the skin and mucous membranes in the gut and respiratory tract become less elastic and resilient with age and so provide a less effective barrier to infection.

Gastrointestinal changes

Changes occur throughout the gut and include a decreased gastric acid secretion in the stomach. In the small intestine the digestive capacity is impaired and in the large intestine there is a decrease in motor function and muscle tone. Diverticula may develop which can become inflamed. The digestive system is therefore more sensitive and susceptible to indigestion and constipation.

Sensory organs

Taste and smell A natural part of the ageing process is a reduction in the number of nasal sensory cells and taste buds. The taste threshold level is increased. As these changes affect taste and smell, the palatability of certain foods is altered. An older person may add more sugar to compensate for the apparent lack of sweetness for example.

Vision Physical changes in the eye can result in astigmatism, decreased visual acuity and diminished colour fidelity. A possible impact is that it is more difficult to see food clearly.

Pain and touch With the reduction in peripheral nerve sensitivity, touch and heat thresholds increase, so for example an older person may hold a hot utensil, not realise the intensity and be burned.

The consequence of these sensory changes is that food may look, smell, taste and feel different.

2 Food – Fulfilling Many Needs

This chapter considers the non-biological functions of food in order to appreciate the wider role of food. It discusses food choice and food selection and identifies the factors that influence our eating patterns. The spiritual significance of food is highlighted as is the impact of religious belief, culture and past experience.

Food associations and needs

Food fulfils many functions apart from meeting the basic need of relieving hunger. Individual foods and combinations of food items remind us of past events and experiences – for example strawberries and cream on a summer afternoon or sponge pudding and custard for school lunch. Foods trigger poignant memories, whether happy or sad.

As well as the biological function of fulfilling our nutritional requirements, food has social, economic, and psychological roles. The psychologist Maslow developed a hierarchy of human needs to explain our individual motivation and how we fulfil our needs (Maslow 1943). This hierarchy has five broad categories which influence how we function. The basic needs are fulfilled before the higher order needs. Table 1 summarises these with food examples.

TABLE 1 FOOD EXAMPLES OF THE HIERARCHY OF HUMAN NEED

Human need	Food example
Basic survival needs – food, water, shelter	Food to relieve hunger
Security needs – physical well-being, protected environment	Sufficient and safe food supply
Group needs – acceptance within a group, sense of belonging, affiliation	A gift of a box of chocolates
Self-esteem needs – to demonstrate success, self worth	Elaborate dinner party or a meal in an expensive restaurant
Self-fulfilment needs – personal development, individual creativity	Food fashion or fad

At a basic level we eat food to survive. If our survival needs are being met, we then move up the hierarchy looking at ways in which we can ensure a safe and sufficient quantity of food. This can be illustrated by some of the activities in the Second World War, and immediately after, where people tended to hoard things. Even now in a food scare you hear of people who have gone out and bought vast quantities of a food for fear that it may not be available shortly afterwards. Over the Christmas period the shops are shut for two or three days and people stock up so that they are not going to run short.

When we feel safe about the quantity and supply of food, then food is used to demonstrate a sense of belonging and acceptance within a social group. Food is given as a symbol of love or affiliation – for example a box of chocolates, a birthday cake or taking food or drink when visiting.

This function of food is particularly important when we are feeling vulnerable or ill, or we are in unfamiliar surroundings. At these times we like to have some familiar food, that has some positive connotations and sense of belonging. This might mean going back to food we have eaten in childhood or food that was prepared and served in a particular way; food that has associations with happy memories.

Moving up the hierarchy, we might use food to show off, to demonstrate social status, wealth and success. When we want to impress people certain perceived high cost and high status foods are shown and used, for example when entertaining.

The final level is when we then want to show that we are individuals and that we are comfortable with ourselves. We may decline a particular food to demonstrate individuality by not conforming with the patterns of food selection normally accepted in our group. It is only when the basic food needs for survival are met, when we feel comfortable and that we belong, that we have the freedom and the ability to demonstrate our individuality.

CASE STUDY 1

Mrs Elizabeth Jones

Mrs Jones sits quietly in the corner, uninterested and uninvolved in her surroundings. She has been in the home three weeks and has not related to any other residents and only communicates with the staff minimally and then with great reluctance.

At mealtimes she has to be coaxed into the dining area and then picks at her food.

The GP has visited and could not identify a physical cause. Although old and frail with chronic arthritis she has no other illnesses and no history of mental health problems.

Q What steps could you initiate to encourage Mrs Jones to relate and eat?

Spiritual significance

Food has spiritual significance in a range of different ways. We give some examples here to help you consider the issues. Be sure to ask your individual clients about their needs rather than making assumptions about their requirements.

Fasting and feasting

Many individuals have their own fasting rules. For example, in the Islamic religion, Ramadan is the month of fasting each year. Within the Christian religion people may fast during Lent. Hindus are quite likely to fast one day a week, or to alter their food intake on particular days of the week. Some Sikhs fast if there is a full moon. It is important to know the fasting rules that govern each individual client, but also those that govern groups of people. These fasting and feasting rules may also impact on seating arrangements.

Special feast days will also be marked by cooking special recipes. One way of acknowledging different cultures and seeking to meet different needs can be by sharing each others' festivals if appropriate.

Food and prayer

People from different religions have particular patterns and times for prayer. For example people following the Islamic religion would want to observe Friday prayers whilst people with a Hindu or Sikh background may have individual patterns that need to be discovered and respected. In lunch clubs and residential settings you will want to be aware of, and be able to accommodate, set prayer times.

Ritual washing

Many religions specify instructions about washing hands and mouths before and after meals. So it is important that the facilities are available for ceremonial washing related to mealtimes. Sometimes a physical disability due to a medical condition, for example a stroke or arthritis, may mean that an individual has difficulty undertaking these activities and so will require sensitive help.

Healing properties

Some individuals and groups of people attribute special healing powers to specific foods. In these instances find out which foods have healing or other spiritual significance to a particular client and either arrange for these foods to be brought in, or enable the person to go and obtain these foods.

Religious issues

Religious belief plays an important role in controlling the type of food we eat, when we eat that food, how we eat, with whom and where.

As more individuals with different religious beliefs require support in the community or enter residential care, an understanding of typical religious food practices is essential so that you can provide appropriate assistance. It is useful to seek permission to contact the client's religious leader (who will be able to provide more information, background and support) as well as discussing needs with the individual client. Some of the religious food practices are outlined below. They are generalised examples – it is essential to ask your individual clients what particular rules they follow.

Islamic food rules

All meat must be ritually cooked and slaughtered (halal). Special prayers are said at the slaughterhouse and all animal products should be halal. Many Muslims will ask for vegetarian food if it is not possible to guarantee that the meat has been ritually slaughtered. Pork, or any part of the pig, birds of prey and the blood of any animal is forbidden. Cooking utensils or serving plates are not acceptable if they have been in contact with pork or non-halal food. Different coloured plates and cutlery can be used to demonstrate that the food has been prepared separately. Food that contains animal fats is not normally eaten.

In many households the men eat first and the women eat later, often in a different room. It may therefore be religiously unacceptable to seat men and women who are Muslims at the same table to eat. The right hand is used for eating, the left for washing the body; therefore a spoon may be preferred to a knife and fork.

Hindu food rules

The Hindu religion stresses the importance of duty to one's family, to the wider society and to all living creatures. Any form of beef is totally unacceptable as the cow is a sacred animal but most Hindus will use cow's milk and butter. Many Hindus are vegetarians who will drink milk and eat yoghurt and curd cheese, but not animal fats such as dripping and lard.

Sikh food rules

Sikhism developed from Hinduism in the sixteenth century and so Sikh food regulations are in some ways similar to Hindu food laws. Many Sikhs are vegetarian and all meat products are avoided. Sikhs do not eat food which has been dedicated to another religion.

Jewish food rules

All meat must be ritually prepared and drained of blood according to specific rules. This is known as 'koshering'. Only meat that has been koshered is acceptable to practising Jews. Cloven hoof animals that chew the cud (for example cows, sheep, goats and deer) are allowed for food but they must be ritually prepared.

Blood and all pork and pig products are totally forbidden. Only fat produced under kosher conditions should be used in baking. Meat and milk cannot be combined in the same meal. So yoghurts for example cannot be eaten as dessert to a meat meal. Different cooking equipment should therefore be used to prepare meat meals and dairy meals. Because of this last factor, many kosher meals are provided in individual frozen portions in foil containers in institutional catering.

Food selection and food choice

Food selection is a complex matter and often over-simplified. In every society some food that is available is not consumed and some items which people eat in another country are considered inedible. For example, frogs legs, which are a delicacy in France, are not commonly eaten in the UK.

Many factors influence our food choice. These factors can be grouped around: previous experience; current environmental conditions; and state of health.

Factors affecting food choice include:

- access
- availability of food
- budgeting skills
- cooking facilities
- cooking and preparation ability
- cooking for self and/or others
- cost of food items
- cultural traditions
- education
- habit
- individual likes and dislikes
- nutrition knowledge
- previous food experience
- religious belief
- state of health
- time of preparation
- willingness to experiment

Webb developed a model for food selection based upon the concept of a hierarchy of availabilities. The factors affecting food choice according to this model are classified into five sequential steps with the decisions made in the earlier stages restricting the later choices (Webb 1995).

The first step is physical availability – if the food is not available we cannot select it. For many older people access to the food is an issue. Is the food available in the local shop? How easy is it to get to the shop and carry the items home? The food might be available in theory but if you have no transport and cannot carry heavy bags you may not be able to do the shopping.

The second group of factors relate to economics and the cost of the various food items. A high proportion of older people (41 per cent) receive State benefits (Finch et al 1998). Is this food item affordable? With a restricted income people's budgets do not stretch to a wide range of food items, especially those that are more expensive. Older people on a fixed income may not be able to afford fresh fruit and vegetables for example.

The next step is cultural acceptance. Would the individual consider purchasing that item? Would they consider it as edible? Cultural availability is affected by our background, our upbringing, our past experiences, our food beliefs, and can be very important, as discussed below.

Fourthly, many people rely on others to undertake their food shopping. In the majority of households the woman does the shopping, and therefore acts as a gatekeeper. She selects the food items and thus makes the choices about which foods are brought into the house. Home care assistants, relatives or neighbours may make similar decisions for an older housebound individual. In residential settings, it is the staff who select the food.

The final category is personal choice, that is the food likes and dislikes of the individual. This is limited by earlier decisions in the filtering process. Therefore the range of food items for personal selection is more narrow and restricted than the range of food that is actually physically available in the locality.

Cultural issues

Culture and ethnicity play a significant role in determining which foods are eaten and how they are eaten. Cultural heritage influences our beliefs and food habits, including food taboos and practices, and must be valued and respected.

People from the Indian sub-continent, those of Chinese origin and those from the West Indies are numerically the most common minority groups in the UK but amongst your residents or clients there may of course be individuals from other cultures and parts of the world – for example from Poland or other parts of Eastern Europe, Cyprus, Greece, or Turkey. All these individuals might have particular requests and particular eating patterns, and it is important that they are understood and accepted. You can ask sympathetically about any food habits and any food likes and dislikes that relate to that individual's cultural background. Friends and relatives or local support groups may be able to give you further information if necessary.

Some typical foods eaten by people from the Indian sub-continent, people of Chinese origin and people from the West Indies are set out in Table 2.

Please remember that these examples are generalised. As we have seen, religious and spiritual factors will also play a significant part in influencing individual requirements.

Further information is available in the publication *In the Minority through the 90's: A handbook for those who provide meals for older people in a multicultural society*. Available from the Nutrition Advisory Group for Elderly People (NAGE), The British Dietetic Association (address on p 120).

TABLE 2 TYPICAL FOODS EATEN BY:

People from the Indian sub-continent	People of Chinese origin	People from the West Indies
Many people from India are vegetarians and their main meals are linked to their staple cereal, which is either rice or wheat depending on which part of India they came from. In southern India it is more likely to be rice. The staple food for people from Bangladesh is polished rice. People from Pakistan consume wheat chapattis or paratha with their halal meat. Rice is served with a selection of other items in smaller dishes of different textures – some thicker, some thinner. Yoghurt, pickle or chutney are served as accompaniments. When available butter, ghee or oil is added to the rice, chapatti and other food dishes.	There are several traditional Chinese staples depending on the crops grown. For example, in some parts of China the staple is rice but further north it is wheat and therefore wheat noodles and wheat dumplings are common. Often the food is cut into bite-size chunks before cooking, saving cooking time, originally because of limited fuel supplies. Many British people think that Chinese food is similar to that served in Chinese restaurants but this is not the case as the restaurants have adapted their menus to accommodate the British palate.	People from the West Indies come from a wide range of cultures, including West Africa, Asia and South America (Venezuela). The staples include starchy roots and tubers, for example sweet potato, yam and cassava. These may be eaten boiled, pounded, dried, or ground into a fine flour and then baked into a bread. Rice, yellow cornmeal and barley are also used as staples. Fish is widely eaten and is either served fresh or processed by pickling, smoking, drying or salting. A wide range of spices and herbs are used, such as thyme for example.

Some people from ethnic groups have integrated into the local population and their general access to food and eating habits are similar to the indigenous population. As they reach retirement age and older their food needs are unlikely to be very different from the majority of the population. Other people still have distinct characteristics which affect their needs in later life.

The extent to which British food habits have been assimilated is influenced by factors such as language and education. Language is particularly important; if an individual does not know the language and has no facilities to learn they can be much more isolated and will have difficulty communicating what they want in shops or restaurants. For example many Pakistani women speak Urdu in the home and their use of English is very limited. If the home-maker is working outside the home, they have more chance to meet other people and come into contact with different foods. They may incorporate some of the new information into their food related activities if they wish.

CASE STUDY 2

Mr Mohammed Aftab

The social worker has visited the residential home to discuss the admission of Mr Mohammed Aftab. She has explained that he was born in Pakistan but has been living in the UK for 35 years. He is Muslim.

Q How would you prepare for his admission?
   What additional factors would you need to consider because of his ethnic origin?

Eating patterns

When we eat is nearly as important as what and why. Our eating patterns are acquired in childhood and subsequently modified in adolescence and throughout our adult lives depending on experiences and circumstances; for example having to do shift work may impinge upon certain mealtimes.

Other factors include:

- cooking abilities
- cooking facilities
- eating alone or with others
- influence of relatives and friends
- living conditions
- previous experiences
- state of health
- time available

Your clients' habits and preferences in terms of eating patterns are thus another element to discuss with them when planning your food services.

3 Nutritional Recommendations and Guidelines

This chapter discusses the current nutritional guidelines and recommendations for older people. It includes information on the current nutritional status of older people based on data from a recent survey and presents information on guidelines for the nutritional content of community and residential meals.

Current nutritional guidelines

During recent years the Government has published documents which provide guidelines for food intake and/or recommendations for the nutrition requirements of different sections of the population.

The current nutritional guidelines for healthy adults are to:

- reduce the total amount of fat, including saturated fat;
- reduce sugar intake by half;
- increase dietary fibre intake by half; *and*
- eat less salt.

In practical terms this means:

- reduce the quantity of fat eaten (found in fried foods, crisps, biscuits, cakes, pastries etc as well as butter and margarine);
- reduce sugar consumption (found in sweets, cakes, biscuits etc as well as that added to drinks);
- increase the amount of cereals and bread (preferably wholegrain), pasta and potatoes; *and*
- increase the quantity of fruit and vegetables. The current recommendation is for five portions of fruit and/or vegetables a day.

These suggestions for changes in our eating habits are based on several key reports, including the Nutrition Task Force (NTF) *Eat Well* reports (NTF 1994; 1995 and 1996) and *The Balance of Good Health* (Health Education Authority (HEA) 1994).

Nutritional requirements

The Committee on Medical Aspects of Food Policy (COMA) has made recommendations for food energy and nutrients for the UK population (DoH 1991). In producing these figures, which are known as Dietary References Values (DRV), for healthy people, the Committee considered that energy and nutrient needs were normally distributed within the population.

They defined four terms:

EAR Estimated Average Requirements of a group of people for energy or protein or a vitamin or mineral. About half will usually need more than the EAR and half less.

LRNI Lower Reference Nutrient Intake for protein or a vitamin or mineral. An amount of the nutrient that is enough for only the few people in a group who have low needs.

RNI Reference Nutrient Intake for protein or a vitamin or a mineral. An amount of the nutrient that is enough, or more than enough, for about 97 per cent of people in a group. If the average intake of a group is at the RNI, then the risk of deficiency in the group is very small.

Safe Intake A term used to indicate intake or a range of intakes of a nutrient for which there is not enough information to estimate RNI, EAR or LRNI. It is an amount that is enough for almost everyone but not so large as to cause undesirable effects.

The energy needs are expressed as the estimated average requirements (EAR) but the nutrients are generally expressed as the reference nutrient intakes (RNI). Table 3 shows the EAR for men and women according to their age.

TABLE 3 ESTIMATED AVERAGE DAILY REQUIREMENTS FOR ENERGY ACCORDING TO AGE AND SEX

Age	EAR MJ (kcal)/day	EAR MJ (kcal)/day
Years	Males	Females
19–50	10.60 (2,550)	8.10 (1,940)
51–59	10.60 (2,550)	8.00 (1,900)
60–64	9.93 (2,380)	7.99 (1,900)
65–74	9.71 (2,330)	7.96 (1,900)
75+	8.77 (2,100)	7.61 (1,810)

(Source: DoH 1991)

In 1992 the COMA report *The Nutrition of Elderly People* (DoH 1992) recommended that the majority of people aged 65 years and over should adopt similar patterns of eating and lifestyle to younger adults in order to maintain health. The report also stressed the importance of maintaining or increasing physical activity to improve muscle tone, muscle power and enhance energy expenditure.

They recommended that all older people should be:

- provided with a diet that is generous in energy (calories). Individuals are unlikely to meet their nutrient requirements when their energy (calorie) consumption is inadequate;
- offered a wide range of nutrient dense foods, ie foods that will provide adequate vitamins, minerals and protein;
- given a diet rich in fibre from wholegrain cereals, fruit and vegetables and with adequate fluid. (Many older people suffer from constipation exacerbated by a low fibre intake. However, in illness bulky high fibre foods may be too filling and prevent someone from eating enough);
- encouraged to increase their intake of vitamin C. As in institutional catering most vitamin C is destroyed, fortified fruit drinks and citrus fruit should be included in the diet daily; *and*
- encouraged to expose some skin to sunlight regularly during the months May to September. Ultra violet (UV) rays from the sun act on the exposed skin to produce vitamin D. The recommended requirement for vitamin D cannot be met from food alone and so

prescribed supplements (see p 80) must be considered for house-bound individuals.

An area of particular concern was the impact of illness and disability on the nutritional status of older people and how a low body weight is common in older chronically ill people. The report encouraged health and social service staff to be aware of the often inadequate food intake of older people and the impact of a poor nutritional status on the development of and recovery from illness (see p 75).

The recommendations of the report about food consumption were as follows:

1	The Working Group endorsed the recommendations for people aged over 50 years in the Government publication *Dietary Reference Values for Food Energy and Nutrients for the United Kingdom* (DoH 1991).
2	Recommendations for dietary energy intakes of elderly people should tend to the generous, except for those who are obese.
3	Elderly people should derive their dietary intakes from a diet containing a variety of nutrient dense foods.
4	An active lifestyle, with prompt resumption after episodes of intercurrent illness, was recommended as contributing in several ways to good health.
5	Steps should be taken to increase the awareness by health professionals of the importance of both overweight and underweight in elderly people.
6	For the majority of elderly people, the same recommendations concerning the dietary intake of non-milk extrinsic sugars (NMES) should apply as for the younger adult population.
7	Intakes of non-starch polysaccharides or NSP (fibre) comparable to those recommended for the general population were advised for most elderly people. Foods with high phytate content, especially raw bran, should be avoided or used sparingly.
8	The statutory fortification of yellow fats other than butter with vitamins A and D should continue, and manufacturers were encouraged to fortify other fat spreads voluntarily.

9   Elderly people should be encouraged to increase their dietary intakes of vitamin C.

10 Adequate intakes of vitamin C need to be ensured for elderly people who are dependent on institutional catering.

11 Elderly people, in common with those of all ages, should be advised to eat more fresh vegetables, fruit, and wholegrain cereals.

12 Elderly people should be encouraged to adopt diets which moderate their plasma cholesterol levels.

13 Elderly people should be encouraged to consume oily fish and to maintain physical activity in order to reduce the risk of thrombosis.

14 The Working Party endorsed the WHO recommendations that 6 grams a day of sodium chloride would be a reasonable average intake for the older population in the UK, and recommended that the present average dietary salt intakes be reduced to meet this level.

15 The calcium intakes of elderly people in the UK should be monitored.

16 Doorstep deliveries of milk for elderly people should be maintained.

17 All elderly people should be encouraged to expose some skin to sunlight regularly during the months May to September.

18 If adequate exposure to sunlight is not possible, vitamin D supplementation should be considered especially during the winter and early spring.

19 Health professionals should be aware of the impact of nutritional status on the development of and recovery from illness.

20 Health professionals should be aware of the often inadequate food intake of elderly people in institutions.

21 Assessment of nutritional status should be a routine aspect of history taking and clinical examination when an elderly person is admitted to hospital.

(Source: DoH 1992)

Current nutritional status

The current view is that if older people are in good general health they should eat the same types of food as the general adult population. Older people on a limited budget are, of course, likely to have a poorer diet with less variety and choice.

A large dietary and nutritional survey of a representative sample of over 1,000 older people (over 65 years) was published in 1998 (Finch et al 1998 and Steele et al 1998). The sample, from across the UK, consisted of two broad groups – people living in institutions and people in the community (called 'free-living'). During the study a variety of techniques were used, including interview, weighed food intake, questionnaires, physical measurements, blood and urine tests and dental examination. Information was obtained about dietary habits, background health status, medication and socio-economic characteristics so that a comprehensive picture could be constructed of the current eating practices and nutritional status of older people in the UK.

Some of the key finding are summarised below, with the differences highlighted between those living in the community ('free-living') and those living in institutions.

The diets of older people

The survey used a four-day food record obtained from nearly 1,700 people to obtain information about which foods and drinks were commonly consumed (Table 4). Potatoes (boiled, mashed or baked), white bread and biscuits were the most frequent food items and tea the most common drink in both groups. Buns, cakes and pastries were eaten by nearly 90 per cent of people living in institutions.

TABLE 4 FREQUENCY OF POPULAR FOODS AND DRINKS IN THE DIETS OF OLDER PEOPLE

Food item	'Free-living' group % consuming the item	People living in institutions % consuming the item
Boiled, mashed or baked potato	87	98
White bread	74	82
Biscuits	71	77
Buns, cakes and pastries	67	89
Wholegrain breakfast cereal	50	50
Other breakfast cereal	28	41
Cereal-based milk pudding	30	89
Other cereal-based puddings	19	72
Whole milk	58	52
Semi-skimmed milk	45	49
Skimmed milk	11	03
Cheese (not cottage)	62	49
Butter	43	44
Polyunsaturated reduced fat spread	29	22
Other reduced fat spreads	13	23
Soft margarine	10	15
Bacon and ham	64	65
Beef and veal dishes	49	74
Chicken and turkey	43	50
Pork	23	27
Lamb	21	37
Coated or fried white fish	36	56
Oily fish	32	34
Other white fish and fish dishes	21	18
Raw tomatoes	52	42

Food item	'Free-living' group % consuming the item	People living in institutions % consuming the item
Salad	47	36
Cooked leafy green vegetables	51	77
Cooked carrots	39	72
Other cooked vegetables	66	77
Chips	44	58
Peas	48	77
Apples and pears	48	25
Bananas	44	35
Citrus fruit	27	12
Table sugar	55	76
Preserves – jam, marmalade	51	69
Chocolates	22	10
Sugar confectionery	06	06
Tea	95	96
Coffee	60	40
Non-diet soft drinks	28	49
Fruit juice	26	14
Beer and lager	19	03
Wine	16	01
Spirits	14	03

(Source: compiled from information in Finch et al 1998)

Accurate information could not be collected about the confectionery and chocolate intake of the people living in institutions, as carers completed the food intake records on behalf of the residents rather than the older person themselves. Nonetheless some notable differences can be seen between the two groups. A more traditional eating pattern is seen in the institutional group. They are more likely to eat non-milk and milk-based cereal puddings and buns, cakes and pastries for example.

The older people who were part of the study were generally adequately nourished. Individuals from three particular groups were more likely to experience problems – people living in institutions, people on a low income and people without their own natural teeth.

The study confirms that older people on a low income are more likely to consume a poor diet than people of a similar age and health but with adequate income. Average energy intakes were lower among people receiving benefits and in the lowest income group. They also had lower intakes of protein, non-starch polysaccharides (NSP) (ie dietary fibre), vitamin C and several other nutrients.

About two-thirds of the free-living group were classified as overweight or obese (67 per cent of men, 63 per cent of women); ie with a Body Mass Index (BMI) – see p 68 – of over 25. One in six of the group living in institutions were underweight (a BMI of 20 or less).

Dental health

As part of the larger survey individuals were asked about their dental health and underwent a dental examination (Steele et al 1998). Overall the people living in institutions had poorer oral health than the free-living group.

On examination they had:

- more unsound teeth
- more unsound crowns
- more root decay
- more new decay
- a greater percentage of plaque
- more unmatched upper and lower dentures sets
- older dentures with more faults
- a lower frequency of cleaning their teeth and dentures

The dental data showed that:

- People with no natural teeth or few natural teeth ate a more restricted range of foods, influenced by their perceived inability to chew.

- There was an association between frequency of sugar intake and decay in those with teeth.
- There was an association between oral function and nutrient intake because people with poor teeth were less likely to choose foods that needed chewing, such as apples, oranges, raw carrots, toast or nuts.
- There was an association between oral function and nutritional status in those without teeth or with few teeth.

These findings suggest the need to pay greater attention to oral hygiene in institutional settings. Specifically these measures should involve: cleaning of teeth and dentures; regular dental check-ups; and less frequent consumption of sugar. There appears to be an association between oral health and general health and so dental care must be given a higher profile across the population.

Food intakes of selected nutrients

PROTEIN

The main sources of protein were (in descending order):

- meat and meat products
- cereal and cereal products
- milk and milk products

The average daily protein intake was adequate for both groups.

CARBOHYDRATES INCLUDING NSP (DIETARY FIBRE)

The main sources of carbohydrates were (in descending order):

- cereal and cereal products
- vegetables, including potatoes
- sugar, preserves, sweet spreads and confectionery

The main sources of non-milk extrinsic sugars (NMES) were (in descending order):

- table sugar
- preserves and sweet spreads
- confectionery

The average daily total sugar intake was above the recommended intake for both groups. Those people in institutions received 18 per cent of their total food energy from NMES instead of the recommended 11 per cent. Older people need to reduce the amount of sugar that they eat.

The main sources of non-starch polysaccharides (NSP) (dietary fibre) were (in descending order):

- cereal and cereal products
- vegetables, including potatoes
- fruit and nuts

The average daily intake was low in both groups, being lower in the people living in institutions (11g for men and 9.5g for women compared to 13.5g for free-living men and 11g for women). The recommended intake is 18 grams a day. Older people need to increase the quantity of NSP that they eat.

DIETARY FAT

The main sources of total fat were (in descending order):

- buns, cakes, pastries and biscuits
- fat spreads
- meat and meat products
- milk and milk products

The average total daily fat intake matched the population average target of 35 per cent of total energy.

The main sources of saturated fatty acids were (in descending order):

- milk
- fat spread
- meat and meat products

Saturated fatty acids contributed about 15 per cent of food energy. This exceeds the recommendation of a maximum of 11 per cent. There is a need to modify the type of fat eaten by older people.

SALT (SODIUM)

Salt was added during cooking by 85 per cent of the free-living group. Salt was usually added at the table by 46 per cent of men and 29 per cent of women in the free-living group and by a higher percentage among those living in institutions (54 per cent of men and 35 per cent of women).

The average intake for both groups was above that recommended and should therefore be reduced.

DIETARY IMPLICATIONS

From this evidence healthier older people should modify their eating habits by:

- reducing the total amount of sugar (NMES) eaten
- increasing the amount of NSP (dietary fibre) eaten
- reducing the amount of saturated fatty acids
- reducing the amount of salt eaten

In practical terms this means:

- avoid adding sugar to drinks
- use wholegrain cereals, high fibre breakfast cereals
- eat more fruit and vegetables
- use semi-skimmed milk
- do not add salt at the table
- use less salt in cooking
- use herbs and spices instead of salt to flavour food

Further information about dietary advice for healthier older people is given in Chapter 5.

Note The information below is still based on weighed food intake but blood samples were taken as well and the blood levels of particular nutrients measured.

Food intakes of selected nutrients (related to simultaneous blood analyses)

CALCIUM

The main sources of calcium for both groups were (in descending order):

- milk and milk products
- cereal and cereal products

The average daily intake of calcium from food sources was above the recommended nutrient intake for both groups. Those living in institutions had a higher intake probably due to the high milk-based cereal pudding consumption.

IRON

The main sources of iron for both groups were (in descending order):

- cereal and cereal products
- meat and meat products
- vegetables

Of the people living in institutions, 5 per cent had dietary intakes which were below the Lower Reference Nutrient Intake (LRNI) and therefore inadequate. From the blood sample 52 per cent of men and 39 per cent of women were classified as anaemic using World Health Organisation (WHO) definitions of anaemia.

VITAMIN C

The main sources of vitamin C were (in descending order):

- vegetables
- fruit and fruit juice

The average intake of vitamin C was above the recommended requirement for people in each group. In the free-living group this average intake decreased with age.

VITAMIN D

The main dietary sources of vitamin D were (in descending order):

- oily fish
- fat spreads
- cereals and cereal products

The dietary intake was below the recommended intake in both groups although supplementation of the diet may be required to achieve the RNI anyway. The best source of vitamin D is sunlight.

Blood analyses showed that 8 per cent of the free-living group and 37 per cent of the institutional group had low blood levels of 25 OHD indicating vitamin D deficiency.

The information from the blood analyses indicated that some individuals were deficient in specific nutrients (Table 5):

TABLE 5 PERCENTAGE OF OLDER PEOPLE WITH A SPECIFIC NUTRIENT DEFICIENCY ACCORDING TO BLOOD ANALYSES

Nutrient	Free-living men %	Free-living women %	Men in institutions %	Women in institutions %
Iron	11	9	52	39
Vitamin C	14	13	44	38
Folate	15	15	39	39
Vitamin B12	6	6	9	9
B vitamin – thiamin	8	9	11	15
B vitamin – riboflavin	41	41	41	32
Vitamin D	6	10	38	37

(Source: compiled from information in Finch et al 1998)

This information implies that an apparently adequate dietary intake of a particular nutrient does not automatically mean that the individual has a sufficient quantity circulating in the blood. Further investigations are needed to discover how particular nutrients are absorbed in the body during ageing.

Guidelines for community meals

The term 'community meal' means a meal prepared and delivered to an individual living in the community. This pre-cooked meal may be served in the client's own home or sheltered accommodation or eaten at a lunch club or day centre. As clients cannot prepare their own meals and can be ill, it is important that the meal provides sufficient energy and nutrients to help in the recovery process.

As many more older people are living in the community, there is an increasing need for community meals and other possible interventions to help ensure adequate nutrition. Resources are finite and the assistance provided must be acceptable and relevant to the client. Adequate monitoring and evaluation procedures help to ensure that alternatives are considered which may be more acceptable and beneficial – such as whether community meals would be more useful in the evening rather than at lunchtime.

As well as the delivery of the food being appropriate, the quality and quantity of the meals must be assessed. Everybody involved – social services department, community meals organiser, volunteers, lunch club providers, catering firms, local restaurants, friends, neighbours – can make informal comments about the food, particularly in relation to taste, smell, texture and temperature. But community meals must conform to a stringent set of guidelines. This will be the responsibility of the care manager, the inspection units or the management teams at social services, and involve environmental health officers as well as the cooks. Your local authority's environmental health department deals with food hygiene and food safety and will be able to provide guidance and details of the appropriate legislation.

Guidelines for the nutritional content of community meals, *Eating Well for Older People*, were produced in 1995 by The Caroline Walker Trust expert working group. As many people receive meals only two or three times a week, the expert working group felt that

TABLE 6 NUTRITIONAL GUIDELINES FOR COMMUNITY MEALS FOR OLDER PEOPLE

Energy (calories)	Not less than 40% of EAR (Estimated Average Requirement)	Women aged 75 & over: 724 kcal (3MJ) Men aged 75 & over: 840 kcal (3.5MJ)
Fat		35% of food energy Women aged 75 & over: 28 grams(g) Men aged 75 & over: 33g
Starch and intrinsic and milk sugars		39% of food energy Women aged 75 & over: 75g Men aged 75 & over: 87g
Non-milk extrinsic sugars (NMES)		11% of food energy Women aged 75 & over: 21g Men aged 75 & over: 24g
Fibre (non-starch polysaccharides or NSP)	Not less than 33% of DRV (Dietary Reference Values)	6g
Protein	Not less than 33% of RNI	Women:15g Men: 18g
B vitamins	Not less than 33% of RNI (Reference Nutrient Intake)	
thiamin		Women 0.3 milligrams(mg); Men 0.3mg
riboflavin		Women 0.4mg; Men 0.4mg
niacin		Women 4mg; Men 5mg
Folate	Not less than 40% of RNI	80 micrograms
Vitamin C	Not less than 50% of RNI	20mg
Vitamin A (retinol equivalents)	Not less than 33% of RNI	Women: 200 micrograms Men: 230 micrograms
Calcium	Not less than 40% of RNI	280mg
Iron	Not less than 40% of RNI	3.5mg
Sodium	Not less than 33% of RNI	530mg
Potassium	Not less than 33% of RNI	115mg

(Source: Caroline Walker Trust 1995)   See Notes on page 34

———— 33 ————

Notes to Table 6 These guidelines provide figures for the recommended nutrient content of community meals prepared for older people over a one- or two-week period. These guidelines are written in terms of nutrients and therefore need to be translated into food items. Two sample menus with quantities are reproduced in Table 7.

Vitamin D – As it can be difficult to supply the full daily requirement of 10 micrograms of Vitamin D in the diet, a prescribed supplement may be needed for some housebound older people (see p 80).

the quality of the food provided must be more concentrated in nutritional terms than a similar meal in a residential home. The community meal is the main meal of the day and therefore should provide at least 40 per cent of the energy, folate, calcium and iron requirements. More details are given in Table 6 on the previous page.

TABLE 7 SAMPLE MENUS FOR A COMMUNITY MEAL FOR AN OLDER PERSON

	Quantity	Food items
Lunch	100ml	Fruit juice
	120g	Steak and kidney pie
	60g	Mixed vegetables
	60g	Cauliflower
	100g	Mashed potatoes
	120g	Trifle
Afternoon snack	60g	Fruit scone
Lunch	100ml	Fruit juice
	100g	Fried haddock
	60g	Peas
	100g	Chipped potatoes
	90g	Bread and butter pudding
Afternoon snack	30g	Shortbread

(Source: Caroline Walker Trust 1995)

Copies of *Eating Well for Older People: Practical and nutritional guidelines for food in residential and nursing homes and for community meals* are available from 'Older People', Broadcast Suuport Services, PO Box 7, London W3 6XJ, price £12.

Guidelines for residential homes

In residential accommodation people depend on others for their food. In many cases all of the food is provided by the home. As the appetite of older people may vary, sufficient food has to be offered during the course of the day to enable clients to meet their nutritional requirements.

The Caroline Walker Trust working party said it was essential that the average day's food, over a one-week period, for people living in residential care, should meet the *Nutrition of Elderly People* report's (DoH 1992) estimated average requirement (EAR) for energy and the reference nutrient intake (RNI) for selected nutrients.

As these guidelines are expressed in term of nutrients rather than in foods, the recommendations have to be translated into food and meals so that an adequate diet can be served that meets nutritional requirements. Recognising this need, the Caroline Walker Trust expert working party commissioned the development of a computer software package. This computer programme is called *Catering for Older People in Residential Accommodation* (CORA) (Caroline Walker Trust 1998) and is designed for anyone involved in planning and providing catering in nursing and residential homes, including the chef, cook, manager or matron. It is easy to use and aims to improve the nutritional quality of food and drink served. The menu planner has over 750 popular and novel recipes from a variety of leading sources.

Using the computer programme menus can be constructed for up to eight weeks to ensure that residents have a mixed and varied diet. The recipes – for all the day's main meals, drinks and snacks – are analysed for their nutritional content. The programme evaluates the food choices and indicates when the recipe selection is inadequate in energy and nutrient content. Alternative recipes are suggested to ensure that the total food offered to the residents meets their energy and nutrient needs. The analysis is based on groups of people and so it will not be able to indicate if a particular individual is eating enough but it will show that a group of residents are being offered sufficient nutrition. It should also help in purchasing and waste control. If you use the package you should be able to demonstrate that nationally

TABLE 8 NUTRITIONAL GUIDELINES FOR FOOD PREPARED FOR OLDER PEOPLE IN RESIDENTIAL AND NURSING HOMES

Energy (calories)	EAR (Estimated Average Requirement) per day	Women aged 75 & over: 1,810 kcal (7.6MJ) Men aged 75 & over: 2,100 kcal (8.8MJ)
Fat		35% of food energy Women aged 75 & over: 70 grams (g) Men aged 75 & over: 82g
Starch and intrinsic and milk sugars		39% of food energy Women aged 75 & over: 188g Men aged 75 & over: 218g
Non-milk extrinsic sugars (NMES)		11% of food energy Women aged 75 & over: 53g Men aged 75 & over: 62g
Fibre (non-starch poly-saccharides or NSP)	DRV (Dietary Reference Values)	18g
Protein	RNI (Reference Nutrient Intake)	Women 46.5g; Men 53.3g
B vitamins thiamin	RNI	Women 0.8 milligrams (mg); Men 0.9mg
riboflavin	RNI	Women 1.1mg; Men 1.3mg
niacin	RNI	Women 12mg; Men 16mg
Folate	RNI	200 micrograms
Vitamin C	RNI	40mg
Vitamin A (retinol equivalents)	RNI	Women: 600 micrograms Men: 700 micrograms
Calcium	RNI	700mg
Iron	RNI	8.7mg
Sodium	RNI	1,600mg
Potassium	RNI	350mg

(Source: Caroline Walker Trust 1995)

Notes to Table 8 These guidelines provide figures for the recommended nutrient content of an average day's food for an older person over a one-week period.

Vitamin D – As it can be difficult to supply the full daily requirement of 10 micrograms of Vitamin D in the diet, a prescribed supplement may be needed (see p 80).

recognised nutritional guidelines are being met in the food offered to your residents.

CORA is available on floppy discs or on CD ROM, price £130, from the Caroline Walker Trust, 22 Kindersley Way, Abbots Langley, Herts WD5 0QD. Tel: 01923 269902. Fax: 01923 445374.

You may wish to seek advice from the local social service catering department when planning your meals. Contract caterers may be able to offer some support but will of course want to provide their own menus. If you wish to use contract caterers, ensure that your specifications are accurate. The local social service inspection unit or the hospital's department of nutrition and dietetics may be willing to advise.

TABLE 9 SAMPLE MENUS FOR RESIDENTIAL ACCOMMODATION

Breakfast	Porridge or high fibre breakfast cereal (150g)	Porridge or high fibre breakfast cereal (150g)
	Toast (white or wholemeal (40g) with butter/ polyunsaturated margarine and marmalade or jam (20g)	Toast (white or wholemeal (40g) with butter or polyunsaturated margarine and marmalade or jam (20g)
	Tea/coffee	Tea/coffee
Mid-morning	Tea/coffee	Tea/coffee
Lunch	Fruit juice (100ml)	Fruit juice (100ml)
	Chicken fricassee (120g) Carrots (60g) Broccoli (60g) Mashed potatoes (100g)	Roast pork (90g) and apple sauce (20g) Cabbage (60g) Sweetcorn (60g) Roast potatoes (90g)
	Apple pie (90g) and custard (90g)	Rhubarb crumble (90g) and custard (90g)
Mid-afternoon	Tea or coffee Jam sponge (50g)	Tea or coffee Madeira cake (60g)
Evening meal	Scrambled egg (100g) Toast (40g) and butter	Fish cakes (120g) and tomatoes (70g)
	Chocolate eclair (45g) Banana (90g)	Cherry pie (90g) Fresh orange (120g)
Bedtime	Milky drink	Milky drink

Daily allowance: 600ml milk and 20g butter or polyunsaturated margarine

(Source: Caroline Walker Trust 1995)

4 **The Service of Meals**

This chapter examines group catering issues. It provides an assessment checklist to help you identify potential difficulties and discusses measures to improve nutritional status at an institutional level, including menu planning and the service and presentation of meals.

Identifying nutrition risk factors

Each residential and nursing home has its own nutritional risk factors. The 'A-Z checklist' developed by Davies is a tool to assist in the process of identification in a systematic manner (Davies and Holdsworth 1979). The checklist could be adapted as appropriate so as to be useful if you are involved with providing community meals. By answering a series of questions you can group the factors into high, medium and low risk, and then highlight the areas of concern and/or where improvement could be made. These can then be prioritised and appropriate action taken to lessen any risk.

A–Z CHECKLIST OF POTENTIAL RISK FACTORS IN RESIDENTIAL HOMES

Every home has its risk factors. Pick out those which apply to your establishment and ask yourself: Why does it occur? Is it a 'high', 'moderate' or 'low' risk to the residents? What steps can be taken to lessen the risk?

A   Weekly cyclic menus or monotony of menu.

B   Difficulties with tea/supper meal menus. (This highlights lack of experience in menu planning and shortage of recipe ideas and may affect costing.)

C Tea/supper meal at or before 5pm. (This frequently occurs, mainly because of staffing difficulties. Biscuits often have to be supplied later in the evening because some residents become hungry before bedtime.)

D Lack of rapport between head of home and cook, or cook resists or resents suggestions.

E Residents' suggestions (for example for recipes) unheeded. Residents' need for special diets ignored. Inadequate committee contact.

F Residents not allowed choice of portion size or poor portion control or no second helpings available.

G No heed taken of food wastage (a large amount of waste indicates a problem).

H Very little home-style cooking. (Residents frequently express desire for familiar foods they have been used to eating, rather than institutional type catering.)

I No special occasion for food treats from the local community or from the home, apart from Christmas dinner.

J For active residents: poor or no facilities for independence in providing food and drink, such as making a cup of tea.

K Hot foods served lukewarm or poor flavouring.

L Poor presentation of food – including table setting, appearance of dining room.

M Unfriendly or undignified waitress service. Meal too rushed.

N No observation of body weight changes of the residents. (Significant changes in weight can be used as an early diagnostic tool for illness, depression or other conditions that can easily affect nutritional status.)

O No help in feeding very frail residents. No measures taken to protect other residents from offensive eating habits.

P Head of home and cook lacking basic nutritional or catering knowledge. Isolated from possible help.

Q Lengthy period between preparation, cooking and serving. Time lag between staff meals and residents' meals, especially affecting vegetables.

R Lack of vitamin C foods or risk of unnecessary destruction of vitamin C and folate.

S	Few vitamin D foods used; combined with lack of exposure to sunlight.
T	Low fibre diet and complaints of constipation.
U	Possible low intake of other nutrients – for example iron, B group vitamins.
V	Preponderance of convenience food of poor nutritional content.
W	Disproportionate costs between: animal protein; fruit and vegetables; and energy foods.
X	Food perks to staff to detriment of residents' meals. High proportion of food served to others.
Y	Conditions conducive to food poisoning. Lack of cleanliness and basic hygiene.
Z	Recommendations may not be implemented.

(Source: Davies and Holdsworth 1979)

These risk factors can be grouped:

- non-involvement of residents
- inadequate menu planning
- poor timing of meals and snacks
- poorly presented and served food
- poorly cooked food
- inadequate food hygiene
- inadequate staff training
- poor organisation within the home

Ongoing monitoring and evaluation of the meal service with consideration of customer satisfaction are important tools. Weight and weight change of clients are useful indicators of the adequate supply of food, particularly energy rich sources. Information obtained from examining menus and from measuring food intake and food wastage should be used in planning any quality food service.

Improving nutritional status

Some of the issues highlighted by the checklist may involve individual changes in practice but others necessitate a broader examination of the organisation. These institutional measures can assist in improving the nutritional status of the residents. They do not diminish the need to monitor individual clients and cater for individual needs but through collating information patterns often do emerge of factors that are affecting several people and therefore require strategic intervention.

Residents' committee

Sometimes older people are reluctant, individually, to voice an opinion, perhaps because they have become institutionalised, accepting the status quo feeling that nothing can change. They may fear rejection and being labelled a troublemaker. This feeling of 'powerlessness' should be tackled in its broadest sense. Everybody should have the right to express a view about their living environment. How would we react if all decisions were removed in our non-working lives?

The formation of a residents' committee can be a helpful step in enabling older people to feel empowered by making suggestions that could improve the operation of their home. Views can also be sought from your clients if you are running a lunch club or day centre for example: the interaction can be of benefit to all. One topic for discussion could be the food and drink provision. Everyone has a view on food so this is a good starting point and could perhaps involve collecting favourite recipes and having a meal chosen by the residents once a week. The topic of food provision should be split for easier discussion and possible action. Possible areas are listed below but the list is not exhaustive nor ranked in any way:

- residents' favourite recipes
- residents' favourite meal
- time that breakfast is served
- variety of breakfast cereal available
- involvement in selecting crockery

- type of flowers in dining area
- type of background music, if any
- celebrating birthdays
- celebrating special occasions
- type and time of evening snacks
- refreshments for visitors
- availability of tea/coffee during day
- meals out
- a bar

Success in a small matter will encourage the group by demonstrating that their views are respected. Some residential and nursing homes now have a snack bar or a small shop where people can buy snacks such as biscuits, fruit, alcoholic drinks, and items such as soap. Other residential homes arrange trips for their more able residents to go out once a month for a meal, or perhaps organise fish and chips every Friday night.

Menu planning

Menus should be planned in advance, in as much detail as possible, and recorded in a menu book, with any changes documented.

Menu planning can help to:

- make ordering easier and more cost-effective
- ensure a well-balanced variety of food is offered which meets the nutritional requirements of the residents/clients
- maintain a record of food served

In planning menus the following practical factors should be considered:

- Give the cook responsibility for the menu planning. Cooks are more likely to be aware of delivery schedules.
- Encourage the cook to talk with the clients about food and their preferences. Clients frequently express the desire for foods they have been used to eating, rather than institutional type catering.
- Encourage innovative ideas from the cook with the agreement of the clients.

- Use food in season, particularly fruit and vegetables.
- Offer a choice of dishes, as variety is important.
- Pay attention to the appearance of the food and the combination of colour and texture.
- Review any menu cycle at least every six months.
- Remember that there will be a wide variation in appetite between residents.
- Ensure that staff do not inflict their own eating habits.

Staff training

All staff need to be aware that the nutritional needs of some older people are different from those of younger people and that good nutrition is an important factor in determining health and well-being. Sometimes a lack of trained staff can lead to the more frail residents not being offered assistance.

As in other areas, staff training needs should be identified and policies and procedures introduced to ensure that these needs are met. This training may involve learning practical skills, such as how to help a frail resident eat, or be more knowledge-based, such as how to meet the particular needs of a resident who has diabetes. Possible nutrition workshop topics could include:

- components of a healthy diet
- how to help a frail resident to eat and drink
- maintaining a food and fluid chart to monitor nutritional intake
- purpose of nutritional assessment
- how to weigh, record and decide when action is required
- stimulating a small appetite
- detecting malnutrition
- what to do when someone decides they do not want to eat
- why, when and how to thicken liquids

Induction programmes for new staff should explain the reasons behind the different policies and clarify the individual procedures as this makes effective implementation more likely, for example with regards to regular weighing of residents to assess nutritional status.

Your local hospital's department of nutrition and dietetics may offer training related to the particular needs of your home or service. The Royal Institute of Public Health and Hygiene (see p 122) runs regional one-day training courses related to nutrition.

Organisation within the residential home

The officer in charge of the home is ultimately responsible for the service provided to the residents. The policies and procedures addressing nutritional issues should be effectively implemented, monitored and evaluated. Issues covered should include the regular weighing of residents to assess nutritional status and early signs of malnutrition, and measuring plate waste as part of monitoring the acceptability of the meals provided.

A key worker could be identified on every shift to take an overview of nutrition issues. Include nutrition related tasks in the job descriptions of various staff so that they are effectively and efficiently undertaken.

Mechanisms should also be in place for obtaining specialist advice when eating difficulties and nutritional problems arise. The staff need to be able to identify when they need a specialist advisor and how they can contact and use that individual or service – for example when and where they can contact the local community State Registered Dietitian or the Speech and Language Therapist (SALT) – see page 90.

Presentation of meals

Factors to be considered in the service of meals can be grouped around the physical environment, social environment and the actual meal. Table 10 lists issues to think about in relation to these headings. These considerations are important as they affect how much food is consumed and how much is wasted.

TABLE 10 FACTORS TO CONSIDER IN THE SERVICE OF MEALS

Environment	Issue
Physical environment	Seating arrangement
	Chairs of appropriate height and type
	Appropriate cutlery
	Noise level
	Distractions
	Avoid offensive odours
Social environment	Sufficient time for eating
	Compatibility of dining companions
	Personal preferences (such as someone who wishes to eat alone)
	Pleasant and non-patronising staff
	Appropriate and discreet assistance
The meal	Portion size
	Appearance
	Taste, smell, colour and texture
	Individual likes and dislikes
	Familiarity and cultural acceptability
	Temperature
	Second helping available
	Sufficient fluid (tea, water, coffee, fruit juice)

(Source: Webb and Copeman 1996)

Physical environment

Try to make the room where the meals are served as similar as possible to an older person's house. The eating area should ideally be:

- a designated place
- pleasant and friendly
- warm
- well-ventilated and draught-free
- well-lit
- free of distractions and unnecessary noise (such as a television)

It should *not* be:

- overcrowded
- congested
- a throughway
- prone to cooking or other odours

Check that the chairs and tables and other furniture are the correct height to allow easy, comfortable eating. Encourage clients who require assistance to get to the dining room, perhaps because they use a Zimmer frame or a wheelchair, to transfer to an ordinary chair for mealtimes; at the very least, ensure that the table is the right height for them to eat meals comfortably.

Small tables where clients can interact while eating are preferable. These should have tablecloths, place settings and condiments and perhaps flowers. Allow adequate space between the tables so that the servers can move easily without disturbing the diners. If particular individuals need aids such as slip mats or wide-handled spoons and forks, an occupational therapist should be involved in deciding the appropriate tools. Ensure also that adequate salt, pepper, vinegar, sauces and drinks are available on the table.

Social environment

Mealtimes are social occasions; to many clients they are the highlight of the day. Take individual preferences into account when deciding dining companions. Some people, perhaps because they are more messy eaters, may prefer to eat alone.

Mealtimes should not appear or feel rushed to anyone. Serve slow eaters first so that they do not feel pressurised if others at the same table have finished eating. A heated plate might be appropriate so that the meal can be eaten slowly and the last bit still consumed at the correct temperature. If assistance is required with feeding, seat the staff member at the same level as the client or resident and offer discreet help so as not to upset them or be off-putting to others.

The meal

You can use either a plated meal service (when the meals are plated centrally and brought to the table) or a family service (when containers are placed on each table and the residents serve themselves from the bowls, deciding for example how many potatoes they want). Whichever is used, clients must feel able to ask for a small or large portion. They should be encouraged to have 'seconds' and not be fearful of having a larger portion than the person sitting next to them. Everyone should have the opportunity to leave the dining table feeling full rather than hungry. Take individual likes and dislikes into account and have alternative food choices available. The meal should look colourful and smell and taste appealing so that it stimulates the appetite. Add gravy and other sauces according to individual taste and ask clients whether they prefer having vegetable dishes and potato dishes on the centre of the tables or not.

Timing of meals

The timing of meals is extremely important. Take clients' preferences into account, including whether they prefer their main meal in the middle of the day or in the evening. If the evening meal is served before 5pm an individual may have to eat all their meals within a seven or eight hour period. Older people often do not eat large meals but prefer to eat several smaller meals.

Some residential homes serve breakfast to each person in their own room. This means that they can take their time over washing and dressing. Residents' preferences in this regard could perhaps be ascertained through the residents' committee.

The provision of adequate fluid is essential. Residents must be offered at least eight cups of liquid during the day. Mid-morning and mid-afternoon drinks should be available as and when people require them. It is useful to have a choice of hot and cold drinks, at any time. More able clients may like to be involved in taking round the tea, coffee and other drinks.

CASE STUDY 3

Mrs Hilda Hulse

Mrs Hulse's daughter has complained that her mother is not getting enough to eat and is hungry in the evening. You chat to Mrs Hulse, a resident, and find out that it is true.

Q What practical steps could you take to resolve the problem? How can you prevent it recurring?

Food preparation

The food provided by the residential home is probably the only source of nutrition – in other settings it is likely to be the primary one – and so it must be adequate. In order to provide nutritious and appetising food, it should be prepared as close to the serving time as possible. Vegetables in particular should be prepared and cooked rapidly, certainly not several hours early. Advice and guidance is available from social service catering and other sources (see p 37).

In any institutional setting the water-soluble vitamins B, C and folate are easily destroyed by heat in the cooking process. They are better preserved by using good quality fresh or frozen vegetables with minimal chopping, minimal cooking and a minimal time-lapse between cooking and serving. High quality frozen vegetables are much better than poor quality fresh vegetables that are delivered to the home only once or twice a week.

Monitor food wastage and ask questions about any wastage, such as whether it is a particular item or a meal that has been rejected and whether the food was poorly cooked, lukewarm or inadequately flavoured?

Suitable contracts should be developed with local suppliers so that high quality raw ingredients are delivered. Finance is of course important but it should not be the prime consideration affecting the food offered. The Caroline Walker Trust expert working party recommended £15 a week should be spent on food ingredients (1994 prices) per resident in residential homes.

The Advisory Body for Social Services Catering (ABSSC) produces *The Catering Checklist* (Biggs 1997), which is aimed at people who are responsible for catering operations but who may not have operational experience as caterers. It covers all aspects of good practice and can be used for training. Further information is available from the ABSSC, tel/fax: 01225 763783.

Food hygiene

The basic rules of good hygiene must be adhered to when feeding older people, particularly those who have reduced immunity and increased susceptibility to infection. Older people are more prone to infections from food and institutions have the potential to cause food poisoning. The three general aims crucial to ensuring the microbiological safety of food prepared for older people are to:

- Minimise the risks of bacterial contamination – ie buy fresh; keep food covered; wash hands thoroughly; use clean utensils, surfaces, and separate chopping boards; and separate raw from cooked foods.
- Maximise the killing of bacteria during food preparation – ie avoid raw and undercooked eggs; defrost thoroughly before cooking; and ensure that meat and poultry are cooked throughout to 70°C.
- Minimise the time that food is stored under conditions that permit bacterial growth – ie prepare as close to consumption as possible; discard food that is past the sell-by date; store leftovers appropriately; and keep food cool below 5°C and hot at 65°C or above.

Your local environmental health officer will have information about basic and advanced hygiene courses and the Royal Institute of Public Health and Hygiene (see p 122) will also be able to advise you on training.

5 Nutrition Issues for Healthier Older People

This chapter examines issues that may be important for healthier older people by looking at conditions which can occur at any age but which are more common among older people. These are constipation, anaemia, obesity, hyperlipidaemia and diabetes. In each case the condition is described and general guidelines on dietary treatment discussed. More detailed information and specific individual therapeutic dietary advice is available from a State Registered Dietitian at your local hospital or health centre.

Constipation

Constipation is a common problem among older people and can be caused by lack of mobility, reduced fluid intake or increased fluid loss. Other possible causes include:

- hypothyroidism (an under-active thyroid)
- dementia
- stroke
- haemorrhoids (piles)
- obstructions in the digestive tract
- conditions which interfere with muscle contraction in the gut
- conditions which alter the fluid levels in the body
- a physical obstruction in the bowel
- a tumour in the abdominal cavity

Prescribed drugs used to treat a variety of medical conditions, from hypertension and ulcers to Parkinson's disease and depression, are also known to have constipation as a potential side effect (two examples are codeine phosphate and morphine).

Constipation is said to occur when someone has difficulty in passing stools or has an incomplete or infrequent passage of hard stools. As the frequency of defecation is very individual (from twice a day to once every three days), an alteration in the normal pattern is significant. People suffering from constipation may feel nauseated and have a reduced appetite. They may experience abdominal pain, a feeling of fullness in the lower bowel and straining as they attempt to defecate.

Treatment

Some health professionals rely on treating constipation with laxatives, suppositories and enemas. The alternative approach to management is to increase fluid intake, ensure an adequate diet and encourage mobility as well as to identify the underlying cause of the constipation and where possible take remedial action.

To treat and prevent constipation, increase the fluid intake to at least eight full cups of liquid (non-alcoholic) a day and increase the amount of dietary fibre, from cereals and vegetables, in the diet.

Dietary fibre is the part of the plant cell wall which the body cannot digest. There are two types of dietary fibre or 'non starch polysaccharides' (NSP) – soluble and insoluble. Soluble fibre dissolves in water and is found in cereals such as oats and vegetables, particularly beans. Insoluble fibre is again found in cereals and vegetables but also in the pips, skins and seed coats of berries for example. It has the effect of holding or absorbing water in the bowel.

Dietary fibre has three effects on bowel function: it improves stool consistency; increases stool weight; and reduces transit time through the colon.

Fibre rich foods include:

■ wholegrain breakfast cereals (such as oats, Branflakes, Weetabix, Shredded Wheat)
■ wholegrain varieties of food (such as pasta, brown rice, wholewheat chapatti)
■ wholemeal bread

- wholegrain biscuits (such as digestives, wholewheat crackers, oat biscuits)
- fruit and vegetables, especially their edible skins (such as unpeeled apples and pears, plums, tomatoes, jacket potatoes)
- pulses (such as baked beans, kidney beans and lentils)
- dried fruit and nuts

Ways to increase fibre intake include:

- Choose a wholegrain breakfast cereal.
- Include wholemeal bread twice daily, for example in sandwiches or for toast. If wholemeal bread is particularly disliked, try a higher fibre white bread such as Champion or Mighty White.
- Include fruit and vegetables daily, eating the edible skins where possible.
- Add fresh or dried fruit, such as banana or sultanas, to breakfast cereals.
- Replace some of the meat in stews with butter beans, kidney beans or other pulses. Try baked beans on wholemeal toast or homemade lentil soup.
- Boil and bake potatoes in their skins. Jacket potatoes are cheap and nutritious.
- Try baking with wholemeal flour. Start by using a mixture of half white and half wholemeal flour in fruit crumbles or scones for example.
- Drink plenty of fluid (not alcohol) – at least 8 to 10 cups daily.

RESIDENTIAL HOME PROCEDURES

People in residential and nursing homes should be offered eight to ten cups of liquid a day. Their actual consumption should be monitored to avoid situations where for example someone is offered a cup of tea but it is removed before the resident has actually drunk it (this may be because it has become cold, it was not placed within easy reach or the individual just forgot it was there).

Toileting arrangements should also be reviewed as some older people are reluctant to drink because they cannot get to the toilet independently or quickly. Clients should be offered assistance to reach the toilet and given as much privacy as possible. Commodes may be quicker but they do not stop other people seeing, hearing or smelling.

A further difficulty is misunderstanding about 'water tablets' prescribed as diuretics. The diuretic works to remove the fluid retained in the body tissues, such as swollen ankles for example. Many people believe that it is beneficial to reduce the amount of liquid consumed when they have been prescribed these drugs but the amount drunk does not have any effect. The purpose of the diuretic and how it operates in the body must be clearly explained – if someone mistakenly restricts their fluid intake they are more likely to become constipated.

Every home should have clear guidelines and a monitoring mechanism for laxative use. The type and frequency of use should be reviewed throughout the home and as part of each resident's individual care plan. This review should be part of an overall policy to reduce the prevalence of constipation.

The Nutrition Advisory Group for Elderly People (NAGE) has a video, *Fibre Keeps you Fit*, which may be useful – see page 120.

CASE STUDY 4

Miss Alison Sutherland

Miss Sutherland has limited mobility and relies on a Zimmer frame to move around. She regularly complains of being constipated.

You notice that Miss Sutherland rarely finishes her cup of tea and other drinks.

Q   When you ask Miss Sutherland about not finishing her drinks, what is she likely to say?
What reassurance and practical assistance can you offer to help her increase her fluid consumption?
When you question Miss Sutherland about her food intake she tells you that she always has cornflakes and white bread at breakfast and

has difficulty eating fruit. How could you encourage Miss
Sutherland to increase the dietary fibre in her diet?
What simple changes in her food selection would be most beneficial
and why?

Anaemia

Anaemia is a common problem affecting many older people.
Anaemia is defined as a state in which there is a low oxygen-carry-
ing capacity of the blood. In measurable terms there is a low
haemoglobin, and/or reduced number of red cells, as well as reduced
packed cell volume (PCV). It is often not diagnosed (recognised)
because the most common symptoms are tiredness, lack of energy,
breathlessness upon exertion and palpitations which are not specific.

There are several types of anaemia with different causes. The most
common type of anaemia is called iron deficiency anaemia. This
occurs when the individual's need for iron exceeds the amount they
are absorbing. This is often due to an inadequate dietary intake or
decreased absorption, perhaps due to a lack of stomach acids. Other
causes include a lack of production of new red blood cells or
increased blood losses. Blood losses can be external bleeding or
internal such as in cancers in the gastrointestinal tract and uterus.

Folate (folic acid) deficiency is another common type of anaemia,
caused by an inadequate dietary intake, malabsorption or
increased requirements.

Treatment

The treatment of anaemia depends upon the cause but improving
the range and variety of food eaten is an important part of treatment for iron deficiency and folic acid deficiency anaemias. Iron
and folate (folic acid) supplements are prescribed as short-term
measures; but in the longer term people should be encouraged to
eat a diet rich in iron and folate. Prescribed supplements should be
regularly reviewed.

IRON RICH FOODS

Iron in the diet comes in two forms – 'haem' from animal products and 'non-haem' from plants. 'Haem' iron is most efficiently absorbed, but the body has the ability to utilise iron from plant sources as well.

Animal 'haem' sources include:

■ offal – such as liver, kidney, liver pâté, liver sausage, black pudding
■ red meat, corned beef, tongue
■ egg

'Non-haem' sources include:

■ fortified breakfast cereals
■ wholemeal bread, wholemeal flour
■ dried fruit – such as apricots, prunes, figs, dates, currants
■ pulses – such as lentils, beans (red kidney, mung, butter, baked)
■ dark green leafy vegetables – such as spinach, broccoli, spring greens, watercress

Ways to increase iron intake include:

■ Use offal and red meat regularly – for example liver and onions, liver and bacon casserole, sauté of kidney, stewed steak and kidney, steak and kidney pie, corned beef or liver sausage sandwich, meat loaf, liver pâté on toast.
■ Choose fortified breakfast cereals.
■ Use wholemeal bread for sandwiches and toast.
■ Add dried fruit, such as apricots, to breakfast cereals and milk puddings or use in scones and other baking.
■ Use lentils, beans and other pulses in soups and stews.

FOLATE (FOLIC ACID) RICH FOODS

The richest dietary sources are:

■ liver
■ yeast
■ green vegetables (especially spinach and brussel sprouts)
■ chocolate

- nuts
- fortified breakfast cereals

Folate compounds are water soluble and are therefore partly destroyed in cooking. In situations where cooked food is kept warm before serving, over 90 per cent of the folate may be destroyed. Good cooking practices will help maintain the amount of folate and vitamin C in foods.

VITAMIN C

Vitamin C enhances the absorption of iron from the gut and therefore it is helpful to eat vitamin C rich food with iron rich food (for example a corned beef sandwich with a tomato). As vitamin C is water soluble it cannot be stored in the body and so a daily supply is needed. It is also destroyed during the cooking process. Fruit and vegetables are rich sources of vitamin C; therefore if older people do not eat fruit and vegetables they are at risk of vitamin C deficiency.

Vitamin C rich foods include:

- citrus fruits – such as fresh oranges and grapefruit
- orange, grapefruit and tomato juice (not tinned)
- vitamin C enriched cordials – such as blackcurrant juice (served cold)
- soft fruit when in season – such as strawberries, blackcurrants, gooseberries
- potatoes (including instant)
- green leafy vegetables (fresh or frozen) or salad

Ways to increase vitamin C intake include:

- Drink a daily glass of fruit juice, or vitamin C enriched cordial.
- Include fruit as snacks or puddings (fresh, stewed, baked or purée). Use a variety of seasonal fruits.
- Cook potatoes in different ways – boiled, baked, jacket, mashed, roast, chipped. Use instant potato with added vitamin C.
- Be careful when storing, preparing and cooking vegetables. Store fresh vegetables in a cool dark place and eat as fresh as possible.

When preparing, wash quickly, as vitamin C is destroyed; do not leave to soak.

■ Cook the vegetables in small amounts of water, for the shortest possible time, with the saucepan lid on.

■ Do not use bicarbonate of soda in cooking.

CASE STUDY 5

Miss Lily Bushell

Miss Bushell is anaemic. The GP has examined her and prescribed iron and folate supplements, as a poor food intake is the likely cause. You are asked to encourage Miss Bushell to increase her intake of dietary iron.

Q   How might you modify the food and drink she consumes?

Obesity

The impact of obesity for older people is similar to that for younger adults but it can also have the effect of dramatically reducing mobility. In many cases active intervention should be considered. Obesity worsens osteoarthritis, heart failure, asthma, arthritis and hypertension, making control of the symptoms of these chronic disorders more difficult.

Obesity is said to occur when an individual's Body Mass Index (BMI) (see page 68) is 30 or greater. Severe obesity is classified when the BMI is 40 or greater. Central obesity, where the excess fat is stored round the middle of the body, including the stomach, is associated with a greater risk of premature death, stroke, diabetes and hypertension than when the excess fat is situated round the hips. Statistically men are more likely to have central obesity whereas women accumulate excess fat round the hips.

Treatment

Effective treatment of obesity is difficult and for many individuals an effective long-term weight reduction programme is hard to maintain. Much research, media interest and scientific debate acknowledges the complexity of the problem but radical effective intervention has yet to be achieved.

Realistic goals in relation to time and weight loss should be agreed. A loss of 1 to 2 kilograms a month is satisfactory and the client needs to accept that a slow steady loss is more likely to be effective in the longer term. A 'starvation' diet is not recommended but regular eating of 'low fat, low sugar, high fibre foods' is encouraged.

Handy hints for weight loss include:

- Eat three regular meals a day and avoid sweet snacks between meals.
- Eat slowly and carefully.
- Avoid fried foods: grill, poach, boil and bake instead.
- Reduce the fat content, by removing visible fat from meat and eating less butter and margarine.
- Change to semi-skimmed milk.
- Cut out sweets, sugar in tea and other visible sources of sugar (for example preserves).
- Drink 'sugar free' squashes and fizzy drinks rather than sweetened alternatives.
- Increase the quantity of fruit and vegetables consumed.
- Eat wholemeal bread and wholegrain cereals.
- Do not feel guilty after an occasional lapse.

Bear in mind that:

- A restricted income will have an impact on the type and variety of food purchased.
- The food provided must fulfil nutrient needs as well as controlling weight.
- Sometimes older people feel it is not worthwhile losing any excess weight.

- Sometimes carers do not feel it is worthwhile initiating change even if the older person wishes to change their eating habits.
- Some people need the support of others and may benefit from a 'slimming group' where they can encourage each other.
- Increasing the amount of exercise and physical activity will assist in weight loss.
- Ill people should not routinely be started on a weight reducing regime.

Hyperlipidaemia

Hyperlipidaemia describes the condition when too much fat is circulating in the blood. There are two types of fat, namely cholesterol and triglyceride. An excess fat in the blood has been identified as one of the main risk factors for coronary heart disease, hence the national health strategy for decreasing the blood cholesterol levels of the adult population (ideally not exceeding 5.2millimol/litre).

The application of this strategy to the older person has not been well established until recent years. The relative risk of coronary heart disease associated with high cholesterol levels declines with advancing age, but the absolute risk of coronary heart disease mortality is greater in older compared to younger people. Older men with a raised cholesterol level are more at risk than older men with a normal cholesterol.

Treatment

Some risk factors for coronary heart disease are unavoidable: increasing age, being male and having a family history of heart disease. Other risk factors are avoidable as they relate to lifestyle, including: smoking, obesity, lack of exercise and a raised blood cholesterol. Once the condition has been diagnosed by a doctor (after a blood test), treatment therefore involves reducing the risk of these lifestyle factors. Stopping smoking and increasing the amount of physical activity are beneficial first steps.

For older people with a raised cholesterol level, there is evidence that a three-pronged nutrition intervention is of value – measures related to weight control, blood pressure and the reduction of cholesterol in the diet. Achievement of a desirable weight and normal blood pressure can have a really marked impact. Specific dietary advice for people with elevated levels of cholesterol depends on how many of a number of variables are abnormal. The overall objectives are to:

- achieve a desirable body weight;
- reduce total fat in the diet to 30 per cent of food energy;
- increase the quantity of complex carbohydrates and dietary fibre;
- increase the consumption of oily fish;
- check alcohol consumption and reduce if excessive; *and*
- modify other lifestyle risk factors such as smoking and lack of exercise.

Ways to reduce the total fat in the diet include:

- Remove the visible fat from meat before eating. Eat lean meat and low fat varieties of burgers and sausages. Remove the skin from poultry.
- Avoid foods with a high hidden fat content, such as crisps, nuts, pies, pastries and chocolate.
- Boil, bake or grill rather than fry foods. When roasting or baking do not add fat.
- Spread polyunsaturated fats or low fat spreads thinly.
- Use skimmed or semi-skimmed milk.
- Avoid cream and full fat milk products. Use low fat yoghurts and other low fat desserts.
- Use small portions of hard cheese (25-30 grams) at a main meal. Do not use cheese as a dessert or between meal snack.
- Eat fish more often, particularly mackerel, trout, herrings or salmon. Choose fish tinned in water, tomato sauce or brine rather than tinned in oil. Do not have fried fish in batter or breadcrumbs.
- Avoid mayonnaise, salad cream, savoury dips and French dressing. Use herbs, spices, vinegar, lemon juice, natural yoghurt, pickles and chutney for flavourings and accompaniments.

These dietary and lifestyle interventions are applicable to fit older people and not to the more frail older person with a limited food intake. Remember that it is quality of life that is important and so the diet should be palatable, acceptable and as near normal as possible. Any proposed intervention must be considered on an individual basis.

The Nutrition of Elderly People report (DoH 1992) recommended that the average person should reduce their salt (sodium chloride) consumption to 6 grams a day in line with the World Health Organisation recommendation. Older people may have a reduced sense of taste and therefore use more salt at the table and in cooking. Herbs and spices to flavour foods could be used as alternatives.

Diabetes

About 3 per cent of the adult population in the UK has been diagnosed with diabetes. Diabetes mellitus is a chronic disorder which affects the body's ability to secrete insulin from the pancreas in sufficient quantities at an appropriate time to enable food to be properly digested and absorbed into the body.

One or more of a range of symptoms develop which cause a person to visit the doctor. These symptoms include thirst, a dry mouth, weight loss, tiredness, lethargy, polyuria (passing lots of urine) and blurred vision. Sometimes no symptoms are present and the patient is diagnosed at a routine health check when a sample of urine is tested and found to contain glucose. There is no cure for diabetes but with effective treatment the individual should live a normal life.

Treatment

Dietary assessment and intervention is part of the treatment of all diabetes but some diabetic patients also need oral hypoglycaemic drugs or insulin. Many adults and older people are controlled adequately by diet and/or hypoglycaemic drugs, but some older people may need to be treated with insulin to achieve good control of blood glucose levels and a sense of well-being.

The aims of dietary treatment for all people with diabetes are to:

■ Achieve and maintain normal blood glucose (normoglycaemia).
■ Achieve and maintain normal weight. Many people with diabetes are overweight and by encouraging them to eat more healthily they are able to reduce their weight and eliminate the primary symptoms of diabetes (thirst, tiredness and lethargy).
■ Prevent long-term complications such as coronary heart disease. People with diabetes have a greater risk of developing coronary heart disease and certain eye problems. Good control of blood glucose levels may reduce the likelihood of these occurring.

The dietary recommendations of the Nutrition Subcommittee of the British Diabetic Association (BDA 1991) can be applied to all healthy people who have diabetes. They recommended that the diet should consist of:

> **Carbohydrate** – 50-55 per cent of the total dietary energy intake, the majority from complex sources (ie foods naturally rich in dietary fibre or starch).
> **Fat** – 30-35 per cent of total dietary energy intake with a maximum of 10 per cent from saturated fats.
> **Protein** – 10-15 per cent of total dietary energy intake.
> (Source: BDA 1991)

If the individual is of 'normal weight' their typical food intake must be appropriate to their energy requirements. When food consisting of more complex carbohydrates is encouraged, there is a danger of an individual becoming 'full' when they have consumed less energy but equal bulk to previous food intakes. This is because the energy concentration of wholegrain cereals, vegetables and pulses is less per unit weight than concentrated sources of energy such as butter, biscuits and cakes. In these situations encourage the individual to eat frequently in sufficient quantities to maintain their body weight, activity level and blood glucose within a normal range.

People with diabetes who are overweight should be encouraged to lose weight by reducing their total energy intake and increasing their physical activity. A slow weight loss of about 1 to 2 kilograms a month is a sensible target rather than a dramatic loss with concurrent loss in lean body mass. Increased physical activity and a more normal food intake of 'healthy' foods should be encouraged. A patient does not need to feel hungry while losing weight.

DIETARY FIBRE (NSP)

The consumption of dietary fibre is an important part of any healthy diet and should therefore be encouraged for diabetic patients. The consumption of fruit and vegetables should be increased.

SUGARS AND SWEETENERS

Obvious sources of highly concentrated sugar should be eliminated, such as sugar in tea or other sweetened drinks such as squashes and fizzy drinks. These provide 'empty calories' rather than any useful nutrients. For people with diabetes who are overweight, eliminating visible sugar can be an effective means of reducing total dietary energy intake. Non-energy artificial sweeteners (such as aspartame and saccharin) can have a role for these patients.

If the diabetic patient is of normal weight the current recommendation is that they should limit their consumption of sugar to that for the general population, ie 25g/day in foods. For many people this would involve a major reduction in the amount eaten.

In recent years there has been discussion as to the merits of substituting fructose for sucrose. Current opinion is that it is unnecessary and that fructose is more expensive and more difficult to use in baking and cooking.

FATS

Altering the quantity and type of fat eaten is for many people the most difficult part of their diabetic control. For many people with diabetes a reduction in saturated fat consumption is important to reduce the risk of heart disease. Saturated fat should only provide 10 per cent of the total energy. As fat is a concentrated source of energy, a small reduction in quantity can have a marked impact on overall energy consumption and hence obesity.

ALCOHOL

Moderate alcohol consumption is acceptable but people with diabetes need to consume alcohol with a meal rather than in isolation. 'Mixers' such as bitter lemon or ginger ale should be 'sugar free'.

Table 11 provides an example of a healthy meal plan suitable for a diabetic patient. The quantity of any particular food item will of course depend on the individual's appetite and activity level.

TABLE 11 SAMPLE MEAL PLAN FOR SOMEONE WITH DIABETES

Breakfast	Wholegrain cereal with semi-skimmed milk Wholemeal bread/toast and scraping of margarine Grilled bacon and tomato if desired Tea/coffee with semi-skimmed milk
Mid-morning	Fresh fruit Tea/coffee with semi-skimmed milk
Midday/ main meal	Lean meat or fish or vegetarian dish Potatoes or wholegrain rice or wholewheat pasta Green vegetables and/or root vegetables Fruit or ½ wholemeal, ½ white flour fruit crumble and custard (without sugar) or low fat dessert (such as a yoghurt) Water or other drink
Mid-afternoon	Fruit or plain biscuit Tea/coffee with semi-skimmed milk
Evening meal/ snack	Cold meat or tuna fish (tinned in brine) or low fat cheese Salad Wholemeal bread with a scraping of margarine Wholegrain fruit cake or fruit or low fat dessert
Bedtime	Tea/coffee with semi-skimmed milk

CASE STUDY 6

Mrs Freda Baxter

Mrs Baxter has suffered from arthritis for many years and takes numerous medications, including steroids. As a result she has recently been diagnosed as having steroid induced diabetes which is not yet properly controlled. She is very anxious about the situation. She is obese (BMI 34) and has a good appetite with a sweet tooth. She enjoys a sweet sherry at the weekend and eats a lot of boiled sweets for her dry mouth. Her daughter often brings diabetic biscuits and chocolate.

Q   **What changes could Mrs Baxter make to her diet and why? How would you help?**
What alternative foods and drinks could her daughter provide?

ILLNESS AND THE OLDER DIABETIC PATIENT

If someone is ill, it is important that they are encouraged to continue eating and drinking. Alternative food and drink items may need to be offered, but a return to a low fat, low sugar, high fibre diet should be achieved as soon as possible. These alternative foods should be easy to eat, not very bulky and pleasant in taste and texture.

Possible alternative food and drink items include:

- tinned fruit and ice cream
- tinned soup and bread and margarine
- rice pudding
- glass of milk and sweet biscuit
- liquid meal replacement (for example Complan, Recovery or Build Up)

For further information about diabetes and older people see the Age Concern Books publication *Caring for Someone with Diabetes* (see p 124). The British Diabetic Association has a Diet Information Service – see page 121.

6 Nutritional Assessment

This chapter describes the nutrition assessment tools available to assess and monitor an individual's nutritional status and discusses factors to consider when using these tools and interpreting the data. Screening techniques for use in the community and on admission to residential care are also explained.

Assessment process

Nutritional assessment means carrying out a series of planned observations and measurements in order to make a judgement about a person's state of nutrition. If inadequate, the cause(s) are investigated to enable a programme of interventions to be designed. This programme may involve dietary advice, social support and/or medical treatment. It may be straightforward, such as providing a wide-handled spoon, or more complicated, such as a combination of community meals, prescribed supplements and better control of a medical condition.

A range of physical (anthropometric) measurements, dietary information, biochemical tests, and visual and clinical observations can be used in assessing the nutritional status of an individual.

Physical methods
Weight

The most important measurement is weight and weight change over time in an individual.

Weight is a measure of the total mass, consisting of the lean body mass, skeletal mass, body fat and fluid. It will change if there is an alteration in the total weight but changes in the relative proportions of the components will not be obvious. As an individual gets older the proportion of lean body mass to body fat is reduced. This means that for the same body weight the individual has less muscle, which will affect their muscle flexibility and strength, as explained in Chapter 1.

The basal metabolic rate (BMR) is the energy the body needs at rest to maintain essential functions such as breathing and circulation of blood. With ageing this is reduced as the body composition changes. As lean body tissue needs more oxygen to function than body fat does, the energy requirements are less. This means that someone who eats the same amount of food is likely to gain weight. Often older people automatically reduce their overall energy consumption and in some situations this means that they are not eating sufficient nutrients and may therefore develop a nutrient deficiency.

When weighing someone, the individual should stand freely, or be seated comfortably, in light indoor clothing on an accurate set of weighing scales and a measurement taken. The weight in kilograms or stones and pounds should be recorded and compared to previous figures. Any changes should be noted and the reason identified. Unintentional weight loss of more than 3 kilograms (7lbs) in three months should be investigated. Ensure that the weighing scales are accessible to all and check them regularly.

PERCENTAGE WEIGHT LOSS

Unintentional weight loss is an important sign of possible disease and/or a change in a client's social situation.

$$\% \text{ weight loss} = \frac{\text{Usual weight} - \text{actual weight}}{\text{usual weight (or ideal)}} \times 100$$

95–100% of usual weight	mild depletion
90–95% of usual weight	moderate depletion
<90% of usual weight	severe depletion

Oedema (retention of fluid by the body) may disguise a weight change and should where relevant be identified.

Height

This is a measure of skeletal size. It has limited value for older people because during ageing curvature of the spine and collapse of the vertebrae may occur, causing some loss in height. Some individuals can lose 5cm in height.

To take this measurement the individual must be able to stand erect, eyes at right angles to the ground. In many cases this may be very difficult because of arthritis. It is often of interest to ask the client their maximum adult height.

Other possible physical measurements are arm span, demispan (see pp 113–114), knee height, skinfold thickness and mid upper arm circumference (MUAC). All involve measuring a part of the body and comparing the result to that expected from standard charts. These charts should be available from your GP or a local community State Registered Dietitian.

Once these physical (anthropometric) measurements have been made, accurate interpretation is important.

Body Mass Index

In the younger adult the weight and height are related in the Quetelet Index or Body Mass Index (BMI).

$$BMI = \frac{\text{weight in kilograms}}{(\text{height in metres})^2}$$

Charts are available so that for a given weight and height it is possible to read off the BMI. Different versions of BMI charts are used and will be available from your GP or local dietitian.

Using different cut-off values it is possible to state if the person is very obese, obese, healthy or underweight.

As the figure obtained involves a multiple of height, this measurement is suspect with older people with skeletal compression. The figure obtained can nonetheless have value in enabling a client to be identified as 'at risk'. For example, a BMI less than 19 should initiate a more detailed nutritional assessment to see whether the client is malnourished.

Dietary methods

The nutrient and energy intake of an individual may be assessed by several methods.

Recall method

A useful technique is to ask the person to recall all the food and fluid consumed during the previous 24 hours. Careful questioning should enable an accurate recall. Remember to ask about any snacks and drinks which may be forgotten. It is important to obtain an estimate of the quantity of each food eaten and the methods of preparation and cooking – for example one slice from a large thin-cut loaf of wholemeal bread or half a medium tomato grilled without any additions. This can get difficult with mixed dishes, such as hotpot or curry.

Possible probe questions about breakfast as part of a 24-hour recall could include:

- What did you have for breakfast yesterday?
- At what time?
- How many slices of bread?
- What type of bread/size of loaf?
- Did you put anything on the bread?
- How much? Can you describe how much – about one teaspoon or two?
- Did you have anything to drink? Tea? In a cup or mug? What size? How many?
- What did you put in the drink? – sugar, honey, milk? How much?

If this 24-hour recall is not typical, more detailed questioning to find out what the client normally eats and drinks is required.

It is also essential to establish if the individual has recently changed their eating habits – for example, if they have been unusually thirsty and drinking a lot of lemonade or fruit juices.

Other dietary methods

Other techniques for assessing food intake are available and are listed in Table 12.

TABLE 12 DIETARY ASSESSMENT TECHNIQUES

Dietary assessment technique	Information obtained
24-hour food recall	What was eaten in previous 24 hours.
Diet history	Typical meal pattern.
Food frequency	How often certain foods are eaten.
Checklist	How often certain foods are eaten (possibly with a score allocated). Used to identify those 'at risk' of malnutrition.
Food diary	Client keeps a record of what they are eating for several days, with details of type, brand and quantity.
Weighed food intake	Before eating anything the client weighs it and writes down the weight. This is very time-consuming.
Food and fluid chart	Type and quantity of food and drinks offered and rejected recorded on a daily chart.

Interpreting dietary information

At a simple level it is important to assess whether the individual is eating regularly and appears to be eating a wide range of food and maintaining an interest in food. Older people are more susceptible to particular nutrient deficiencies if their overall energy intake appears low. Using a checklist or scoring system has advantages as it can enable a rapid assessment.

In the residential setting a food and fluid chart (see pp 86–87), client likes and dislikes and portion size are usually the most useful pieces of dietary information to collect.

Biochemical tests

Biochemical tests should not be used in isolation but to complement a verbal and visual assessment of the individual. Laboratory tests may include routine serum nutrient levels, white and red blood cell levels or more specific investigations of urinary or faecal losses. They can be useful in detecting subclinical malnutrition (ie an 'early warning') but the results must be interpreted with care.

Visual observations

The observation of an individual, perhaps with loose fitting clothes and an emaciated appearance, may trigger off further investigations into their nutritional status, but on occasions it can be overlooked, if dismissed as an automatic part of a disease or the ageing process.

Remember that it is possible to be overweight and malnourished, particularly for older people. Typically the individual who is over-weight at 80 years was overweight at 45 or younger. As their food intake matched their energy expenditure, they maintained their excessive weight. As they have become less active, some individuals may have reduced their food intake. Consequently their current food intake may be inadequate to provide sufficient nutrients to meet the body's requirements, particularly of protein and some of the water soluble vitamins.

Clinical observations

A full physical examination of an individual may reveal muscle wasting, oedema (retention of fluid in the body) and other clinical signs of malnutrition. It is important that a medical and drug history is obtained to assess the possible causes and to enable appropriate intervention. During the course of the physical examination it is useful if the doctor or nurse enquires about social circumstances. In many situations, changing social and economic circumstances can have a profound effect on the nutritional status of an individual.

CASE STUDY 7

Mrs Anila Khan

You suspect that Mrs Khan is losing weight as you have noticed that her clothes are hanging more loosely.

Q   What steps would you take to check her weight?
What mechanisms should be in place to ensure that any changes in weight in the residents are noted and the causes investigated?

Nutrition screening

Screening is a method of identifying those who are 'at risk', so that appropriate, relevant interventions can be designed and implemented. The term screening when applied to older people includes the notion of screening for disability as well as for clinical and sub-clinical disease.

Nutritional screening seeks to identify those who are 'at risk' of under-nutrition or over-nutrition or a nutrition imbalance. The initial screening can be conducted by neighbours, relatives, home care assistants or the older person themself.

The basic idea is to consider social and environmental factors which may make a person susceptible to malnutrition and relate these to their current health status and food intake. Social, biological or environmental circumstances could include being housebound, living alone, chronic bronchitis or poor teeth or dentures. This does not mean that everybody who is housebound for example is mal-nourished, but it is a risk factor that could contribute towards malnutrition.

Current health status and food intake factors may include a recent weight change, higher alcohol consumption, missed meals, insufficient food stores at home or an acute episode of illness. These all mean that the vulnerable person is more prone to malnutrition. Early identification and action can often prevent further deterioration and loss of quality of life.

Nutrition screening tools

Many health professionals have developed screening tools which are easy to use either on admission to hospital or other residential setting or in the person's own home.

Most screening tool questionnaires about nutrition include questions related to:

- current food intake
- recent weight change
- appetite
- swallowing
- medical and physical condition including medication
- mental/socio-economic state

Some screening tools have a scoring system which allows the nurse or other health professional to refer the 'at risk' client, whose score is outside the acceptable range, for more advice and assistance. Some screening tools have more than one outcome depending on the score; this can include additional food supplements for a less abnormal score.

The Nutrition Advisory Group for Elderly People (NAGE) of the British Dietetic Association produced a nutrition assessment checklist in 1990 (see p 120 for details). It is likely that the department of nutrition and dietetics at your local hospital or your community dietitian will have a screening tool which is used locally.

Nutrition screening on admission to residential care

Assessing the nutritional status of an individual entering residential care is essential. One officer in charge of a residential home has said: 'It is only when a new resident starts to eat properly that I know they are beginning to accept the situation and adapt to their new sur-roundings.' The assessment should be conducted in a systematic, empathetic manner to enable the individual to feel that they are able to give appropriate and accurate answers.

At the initial interview it is important to find out from the client:

- Current weight and any recent weight change. Loose fitting clothes or a belt on a different notch can suggest a weight loss. (But check that they are the client's usual clothes.) This measurement is particularly helpful as it gives a standard against which future progress or decline can be measured.
- Appetite – is it normal and, if not, for how long has it been altered?
- Habitual food intake, meal patterns, food likes and dislikes including details of snacks eaten.
- Any particular supplements taken, whether prescribed or bought over the counter (such as cod liver oil).
- Details of any medicines whether prescribed (such as steroids) or bought over the counter (such as laxatives). Many drugs interact with an individual's appetite or affect the absorption and utilisa-tion by the body of particular nutrients.
- Any special dietary requirements for cultural, religious, or thera-peutic reasons.

It is important to continue to build up a picture of the new resident's dietary habits and needs over the first few days. A food and fluid intake chart may be of value initially (see pp 86–87). What was the prime reason for the admission? A sudden deterioration in physical and/or medical condition; or the culmination of many weeks of planning related to a broader social situation? The loss of a spouse and giving up of a home are traumatic life events and often cause depression and a temporary loss of appetite.

Malnutrition

A study in 1994 indicated that over 40 per cent of older people admitted to hospital are malnourished and this percentage increased during their time in hospital, so that by discharge 76 per cent of people were malnourished (McWhirter and Pennington 1994). Other studies have confirmed these findings. In 1996, in response to complaints from patients' relatives and media coverage about older people 'starving in hospital', the Department of Health commissioned a resource for improving dietary care in hospitals (Bond 1997) for all NHS trusts in England. This resource acknowledges that hospital admission can have a dramatic effect on how well a patient eats and drinks relative to their individual needs.

Malnutrition occurs when the body has insufficient food to meet its physiological and activity requirements. The balance between food intake and energy and nutrient expenditure can be disturbed by an increase in requirements, such as during an acute or chronic illness, or by a reduction in food and drink consumed. Energy requirements are increased because the metabolic rate is raised in illness, for example by surgical trauma, burns, cancers, infection or fractures.

In hospital and other institutions many factors influence someone's inclination and ability to eat. These include physical difficulties, dislike of food offered, loss of appetite due to illness, side effects of drug therapy or missing meals due to tests and other medical procedures.

As well as malnutrition and an increased risk of death, a poor nutritional status can have a marked impact on the recovery process. The consequences of a poor nutritional status can include:

- higher rate of wound infection
- increased risk of general infection
- increased risk of pressure sores
- increased liability to heart failure
- increased likelihood of a range of adverse psychological conditions, such as apathy or depression.

A recent enquiry commissioned by the Department of Health into the care of older people in hospitals across England (Health Advisory Service 2000 1998) found that the lack of flexibility in hospital routines meant that people were left without food and drinks for long periods of time. The interpretation of the Health and Safety regulations meant that some people were not allowed to have their particular food choice even if a relative wished to bring in the item. Relatives frequently reported a lack of help from staff in relation to feeding. Staff did not always recognise or respond to people who needed help with reaching or eating their food. There was also uncertainty about who was responsible for ensuring patients achieved adequate levels of nutrition and there was a lack of under-standing about more specialist areas, such as swallowing assessments after a stroke. The subsequent Health Circular said that these findings were unacceptable and that as a minimum 'older people must expect to receive the essentials that underpin recovery in hospital; to be well nourished, clean, dry and comfortable and to be treated with due respect'. Practices and procedures within any residential setting caring for vulnerable older people should be examined in the light of these findings and the statement in the Circular.

7 Tackling Eating Problems

This chapter suggests how to stimulate a small appetite and how and when to use food supplements. It also provides suggestions on ways to help someone who is having difficulty in swallowing consume sufficient food and fluid.

Stimulating a small appetite

When people are ill their appetite is often impaired. They may feel apathetic about preparing food or nauseated by the sight and smell of food. The food may taste of 'cardboard' or it requires too much effort to take the food from the plate to the mouth or even chew the food. This may be due to the illness itself and/or the medication.

If someone is adequately fed immediately prior to an acute illness they have sufficient food stores for a few days, but if someone is only marginally nourished, recently discharged from hospital or previously only ate a small variety of foods they are much more susceptible to malnutrition. As malnutrition delays the recovery process it is important to consider ways to persuade someone to eat more – to stimulate a small appetite.

The initial step is to identify any specific problems, such as a physical difficulty in handling cutlery or a dry or sore mouth. Possible reasons for a poor appetite include:

- changing sense of taste and smell
- constipation
- dry mouth
- ill-fitting dentures

- lack of motivation
- mouth infection
- physical difficulty handling cutlery

Ill-fitting dentures or a mouth infection, such as thrush or ulceration for example, may cause a sore mouth. Very sour foods such as lemons and other fruit or very hot foods will aggravate this pain and should be avoided until the mouth infection is treated.

A dry mouth is often a side effect of medication or illness. Fizzy drinks before a meal can refresh the mouth, and chewing ice cubes can stimulate saliva production. If necessary artificial saliva can be prescribed which will enable the person to lubricate their food.

Prescribed and non-prescribed drugs can alter the appetite and consequently affect the amount of food consumed. It is useful to maintain a list of the potential side effects of the commonly used prescribed and non-prescribed drugs.

It is helpful to explain to the person and their carers the importance of good nutrition in their recovery as it may increase their motivation to try and eat their meals and to drink adequately.

Further information is available in the NAGE publication *Taking Steps to Tackle Eating Problems: A handbook and poster for those who care for older people* (see p 120).

Sensitive help with feeding

The points made in Chapter 4 (see pp 44–47) about the presentation of meals are relevant with regard to making mealtimes enjoyable occasions and not an ordeal for the client with a small appetite.

The following additional hints may also assist:

- Do not undertake messy procedures immediately before a meal.
- Seat the person comfortably in an upright position, supported where necessary by additional pillows or cushions.
- Make meals a social event by encouraging the person to sit at a table with others.

- Pay attention to the presentation of the food so that it looks appetising and the portions are not so large as to be off-putting.
- Ensure that the food is within reach of the person and that any necessary feeding aids are provided.
- Offer a small glass of sherry, brandy or beer before a meal as this can be an excellent appetite stimulant (provided it is medically acceptable).

CASE STUDY 8

Mr John Godfrey

Mr Godfrey, a resident of several months, has always been a steady eater. He is recovering from a recent illness and unfortunately now has no appetite and is reluctant to eat.

Q How could you stimulate his appetite and improve his food intake?

If assistance is required it should be provided in a sympathetic, supportive manner which ensures dignity and does not create unnecessary dependence. The following points may be helpful in this respect:

- Check equipment and posture before the meal arrives.
- A helper should only assist one client at a time.
- The helper should sit in the client's eyeline.
- Check the seasoning. Add sauces and condiments to the client's taste.
- Be patient. Food should be offered at the client's natural rate of eating.
- Make sure that the food is maintained at an appropriate temperature throughout the meal.

Rejecting food

It can be difficult to care for someone if they keep changing their mind about what they want to eat. It is important not to feel guilty.

Remember that rejecting food may be the only way an individual has of exerting any control on their environment and so have alternatives available.

Medication, particularly chemotherapy, can dramatically alter someone's perception of taste and smell and interfere with the production of saliva in the mouth, making food taste like cardboard. Other people may be reluctant to eat or drink if they have no sense of thirst or hunger or if they cannot remember if they have eaten or not.

Nourishing snacks throughout the day and early evening may be a solution, particularly if they are small and easy to hold. Some individuals may find single texture meals helpful. Cornflakes with cold milk is multi-textured and thus is more difficult to eat than porridge oats/Ready Brek for example.

Supplements

A nutritional supplement is an item given in addition to the ordinary diet to increase the energy and/or nutrient value. There are several types of supplements.

'Little and often' – a snack

It may be possible to increase someone's nutritional intake by offering small quantities of food at frequent intervals throughout the day and evening. For example a milky drink mid-morning and a piece of cake in the middle of the afternoon as snacks in addition to the normal meals. But make sure that the person does not feel overwhelmed with too much at any one time.

Small nourishing snacks can be helpful for small appetites. You could try:

- cheese and buttered crackers
- sandwiches, white or wholemeal, with a quality protein filling such as egg, ham, cheese, tuna or corned beef
- whole milk yoghurt and other full cream dairy desserts
- toasted currant teacake and a glass of milk
- scone with butter and jam

- bedtime drink, such as Horlicks, cocoa or Ovaltine, made with the correct quantity of full fat milk

Enriched food

If people are only consuming a small quantity of food, every mouthful must count in terms of energy and nutrients. The nutrient value of food can be increased by adding other food items which do not increase the bulk of the original food.

Possibilities include:

- butter or margarine added to vegetables and potatoes or spread thickly on bread, toast, crackers or scones
- jam, honey, syrup or marmalade added to milk puddings or spread generously on bread, toast or crackers
- double cream and evaporated milk added to porridge, puddings, soups, sauces and fruit
- sugar added to drinks, breakfast cereals, fruit and puddings
- salad cream added to sandwich fillings such as tuna or well-cooked eggs
- grated cheese sprinkled on top of cooked vegetables, potatoes, soups, sauces and fish

Milk can be fortified with milk powder and the 'fortified milk' used in place of ordinary milk throughout the day. The normal recipe is to add 2 heaped tablespoons (60g) of milk powder to 1 pint full fat milk and mix well. This will double the protein and increase the energy content. Once made, it should be labelled with the date, and kept covered in the fridge. (After 24 hours any unused 'fortified milk' must be discarded.) This milk should be used for drinks such as coffee, Horlicks, Ovaltine and drinking chocolate, on breakfast cereals and porridge, in soups and sauces, and in puddings such as jelly, custard and milk pudding. One tablespoon of milk powder per portion can be added to soup, milk pudding, custard or porridge if there are only one or two people needing extra protein.

The meal plan guide in Table 13 offers some suggestions as to how and when food can be enriched throughout the day. Remember not to offer too large a portion as small portions served attractively are more likely to stimulate a person's appetite.

TABLE 13 SAMPLE MEAL PLAN FOR OFFERING SNACKS AND ENRICHING FOOD

Mealtime	Possible food items	Ways to enrich the food offered
Early morning	Tea and biscuits	Use fortified full fat milk
Breakfast	Fruit juice Porridge or breakfast cereal	Use fortified milk, add sugar
	Cooked breakfast eg bacon and tomatoes, scrambled egg	
	Bread or toast with butter and jam or marmalade	Generous serving
Mid-morning	Coffee	Milky coffee
	Biscuit or sliced fresh fruit	
Lunch	Meat, chicken, or fish	
	Vegetables	Add grated cheese or butter
	Potatoes	and fortified milk
	Sponge with custard	Use fortified milk
	or milk-based pudding	Add jam or honey
	or fruit crumble with evaporated milk	Full cream
Mid-afternoon	Tea or coffee	
	Cake or scone with butter	Spread generously
Evening meal	Soup	Add cheese, diced cooked meat, lentils, or cream
	Macaroni cheese or sandwiches – eg ham, tuna, cheese, hard-boiled egg	Add salad cream, mayonnaise or chutney
	Mousse or tinned fruit or jelly and ice cream	Use fortified milk
Bedtime snack	Milky drink	Use fortified milk
	Biscuit or crackers with cheese	

Supplementary products

Supplementary products are available from the pharmacy and may be commercially available (such as Complan or Build Up) or prescribed (such as Fortisip or Ensure). They are designed to give extra protein, energy and other nutrition in powder, liquid or dessert form. The products supply a range of different nutrients and come in a variety of sweet and savoury flavours. The puddings are generally smooth ready-made desserts that are energy-rich and nutrient-rich.

The powders are predominately sources of energy being carbohydrate sources. These are generally dextrin or maltose and are less sweet than sucrose and therefore do not change the taste of a particular food. They are sprinkled onto ordinary food and stirred in or dissolved in water or another liquid and the resulting sweetened liquid used. Common products include Maxijul, Caloreen and Polycal.

WHEN TO USE SUPPLEMENTARY PRODUCTS

Many medical conditions allow these products to be prescribed but check with the doctor that there is no secondary medical reason to prevent their use. They are not designed to be the total source of nutrition or a food substitute but to supplement a small food intake. They can be used occasionally to replace an uneaten meal or more systematically to increase the total energy and nutrient intake.

Supplementary products can be useful:

■ to increase the nutrient intake of a client with a restricted diet;
■ to supply extra nutrients for clients who have an increased need (for example to help wound healing or while fighting an infection); *or*
■ to increase the nutrition of those who only eat a small range of foods.

SERVING SUGGESTIONS

Offer the client a choice from the many products available. Ask your client if they would prefer the products at mealtimes or between meals. You should usually offer two or three supplements daily. These could include:

■ Savoury drinks and soups – heat gently, but do not boil. Serve in a bowl or mug with crackers, toast or a bread roll.

■ Sweet drinks – identify the serving temperature most acceptable to the client. Some are served in small cartons (tetra packs) with a straw and can be consumed direct or they can be decanted into a glass and served chilled or warmed depending on the preference. If serving hot, heat gently and do not boil as this changes the taste. For ice cream or sorbet, freeze it in the package or follow the manufacturer's recommendations. You can also use it as a sauce to pour over ice cream or tinned fruit.

■ Puddings – these can be served chilled on their own, with fruit, ice cream or with sponge fingers.

Recipe booklets are available from the manufacturers to show how the supplement can be used in a variety of ways in foods and in drinks in a person's diet. Select products that are acceptable and palatable to your client. Before using any product check that the packaging is not damaged and that the use by date has not expired. Any opened product should be discarded within half a day.

MONITORING SUPPLEMENTARY PRODUCTS

The use of supplements should be monitored and a regular review system agreed.

The following factors should be taken into consideration:

■ type of supplement required (ie energy source and/or other nutrients)
■ likes and dislikes of patient
■ milk or non-milk supplement
■ quantity of supplement prescribed
■ quantity of supplement consumed
■ total fluid consumed
■ concurrent intake of ordinary food

The impact of the supplement on other food and fluid consumed should be recorded for each individual. A potential danger is dehydration if the total fluid intake is not monitored because many supplements have a high energy concentration and some older people consume a supplement drink instead of a normal drink.

Encouraging fluids

Mild dehydration is a common problem among older people and can cause electrolyte imbalance in the body and sometimes confusion. As part of the ageing process the sense of thirst and the ability to react to temperature changes (homeostatic regulation) are reduced. This means that older people will not feel thirsty as quickly as younger people in the same situation and that their bodies take longer to correct any water imbalance.

Reluctance or inability to drink can be due to a variety of factors (Table 14). These can be related to health status, psychological influences and practical obstacles.

TABLE 14 FACTORS THAT MAY RESULT IN A LOW FLUID CONSUMPTION

Immediate reason	Possible cause
Restricted mobility	arthritis, frail
Cannot grip cup	arthritis
Cannot lift cup	stroke
Cannot lift cup to mouth	lack of co-ordination hand to mouth
Sore mouth	infection, drug side effect, chemotherapy
Swallowing difficulty	stroke, Parkinson's disease
Fear of incontinence	previous experience
No interest in drinking	depressed
On 'water tablets'	therefore thinks must drink less
Not offered drink	routine at home or day centre
No free access to drinks	routine (eg no water jugs) at home or day centre
Drink not placed within reach	carer not aware of individual client's needs
Type of drink given not liked	individual preferences not considered
Temperature of drink	lukewarm tea – poor routine
Inadequate toileting arrangements	poor routine – resident does not feel able to ask
Side effect of drug	interaction with drugs, disease state
Feels 'bloated'	constipation
Not encouraged to drink	does not feel thirsty – poor routine

Any intervention must be based on an accurate assessment of the reasons for a low fluid intake. It is helpful as a first step to consider your own fluid consumption. List all the drinks you have in 24 hours, noting the type, quantity and context. An example is given in Table 15: compare this with the amount offered to the residents.

TABLE 15 SAMPLE LIST OF DRINKS CONSUMED IN 24 HOURS BY A CARER

Time	Drink	Context
7.00am	mug of tea, glass fruit juice	at home
8.30am	cup of tea	arrived at work
10.30am	mug of coffee	break
1.00pm	2 cups of tea	lunch break
3.30pm	cup of tea	afternoon break
5.30pm	mug of coffee	preparing meal
7.00pm	mug of coffee	with evening meal
during evening	pint lager, 2 tonic water	at pub
11.00pm	milky drink	before bed

Remember that you have only listed the number of drinks, not the total fluid consumed. Many foods are partly liquid and therefore provide an additional source of fluid. For example custard and gravy are obvious liquids but meat and vegetables, depending on how they are cooked, can contain a significant percentage of water.

Total fluid input should average about 2,500 ml a day in order to maintain the fluid balance in the body. Therefore a suggested intake is between eight and ten cups a day of non-alcoholic liquid.

You can monitor the situation using a food and fluid intake chart. The key worker, or if they are not available, a designated staff member for every shift, should have the responsibility for monitoring and ensuring that an accurate record is obtained for a particular client. Record the actual amount consumed, not that offered. A partly completed example is given in Table 16.

TABLE 16 SAMPLE FOOD AND FLUID CHART

Time	Food/fluid offered	Food/fluid eaten	Waste	Checked by (initials)
7.00am	1 cup of tea (180ml)	half drunk	half	JPC
9.00am	1 Weetabix + milk	all	–	JPC
	1 buttered toast + teaspoon jam	all all		
	1 cup of tea + 1 cup of tea (refill)	all all		
10.30am	1 cup of milky coffee	quarter	three-quarters	JW

Day 7th May

Name of Client Alan Jones

Other non-oral sources of fluid (eg intravenous drip) None

Once it has been established that there is a low fluid intake the reasons should be ascertained and appropriate action taken. Some individuals will need coaching to drink, and, if their memory is impaired, reminding to drink. Others may need physical assistance or the liquid thickening. Some of the more able residents may wish to make their own drinks as desired. Other causes will require a review of the home routine as they are beyond the scope of the carer - for example if lukewarm tea is being offered.

Training programmes for staff will increase awareness and improve knowledge but appropriate procedures and monitoring must be introduced by the management for some causes to be effectively eliminated. Look at organisational issues such as how often the residents are offered drinks and mechanisms to ensure that each individual has the drink of their choice.

CASE STUDY 9

Mrs Irene Morgan

Mrs Morgan has had a stroke which means that she has limited movement on her left side. She can only lift her left arm a few inches and cannot hold anything in it. She also has difficulty communicating.

Q **What likely eating and drinking difficulties will she experience? What practical assistance could you give to help reduce their impact?**

Swallowing difficulties

Dysphagia is the medical term for a difficulty in swallowing. The clinical signs of dysphagia are:

- chest infection
- chronic congestion
- coughing/choking on food or drink
- inability to swallow voluntarily
- poor or absent cough reflex
- poor chewing ability
- refusal to eat certain foods
- regurgitation of food and/or drink
- weight loss
- wet or gurgly voice quality

Obviously not everyone experiencing these signs has an abnormal swallow – for example weight loss has many other causes - but a combination of these signs should justify further investigation.

Not all patients with dysphagia have obvious signs. If a problem with swallowing occurs it is important that a Speech and Language Therapist (see p 90) makes an assessment to identify the specific difficulty and the precise location. The normal swallow action can be divided into three stages: when the food is in the mouth (oral);

the actual swallow (pharyngeal); and the movement of the food down the oesophagus into the stomach (oesophageal).

Problems in the mouth (oral phase) include:

- an inability to close the lip
- limited tongue control
- reduced chewing
- a loss of sensation
- an inability to clear the residue

If the lip cannot close properly, soft food and liquids will dribble out of the mouth causing discomfort, embarrassment and a reduced fluid intake. Limited tongue control and the reduced ability to chew means that the food is not made into a bolus (soft ball) easily. A lack of saliva may compound this effect.

The most common difficulty in the pharyngeal phase is an inadequate swallow reflex leading to nasal regurgitation and/or entry of food into the airway. This occurs when the 'flap' at the back of the mouth does not close quickly enough and the food and fluid, instead of entering the oesophagus and stomach, go into the trachea and lung. If this happens to a healthy person, they cough to remove the foreign food from the lung. When someone is experiencing difficulty swallowing, this normal cough reflex action is inhibited.

Problems in the oesophagus are rarer. When they do occur they are often due to a blockage, growth or physical narrowing which may require surgical intervention.

It is estimated that 50 per cent of people with Parkinson's disease experience difficulty with swallowing. Typical swallowing problems associated with the disease include tongue pumping and delayed reflex. Many sufferers have problems with chewing and manipulating the food in the mouth. Because of rigidity of the muscles in the mouth and in the surrounding areas, often when the food enters the mouth the tongue goes forward and so the individual experiences difficulty forming a bolus with the food.

About 30 per cent of stroke patients have an abnormal swallow initially. By day seven the figure is still as high as 15 per cent. Patients may experience a reduced ability to chew certain foods, incomplete lip closure with dribbling, or an inability to manipulate the tongue. A diminished facial sensation on one side of the mouth may mean that food is pouched. Lack of saliva production means that the individual cannot form a bolus with their food.

The consequences of dysphagia may be short-term, such as dehydration and aspiration, or, in the longer term, malnutrition. If not diagnosed and treated promptly it can affect the recovery rate and chances of long-term disability in an individual.

As part of the initial assessment of a person with swallowing difficulty the Speech and Language Therapist (SALT) should assess the individual's swallow and identify where the difficulty is. Decisions about which textures to use should be made once this assessment has been discussed. SALTs are based either at the hospital or in the community and can be contacted through your GP.

Feeding a patient with dysphagia

The goal in feeding an individual with dysphagia is to maintain or improve nutritional status and to ensure safety during feeding.

Many people with swallowing impairment find it easier to concentrate on a single texture. To facilitate choice, food can be categorised in terms of texture and the ease of consumption. One classification divides food textures into challenging and easier foods, as shown in Table 17.

The classification reflects the importance of the thickness or thinness of a food and texture combinations. For example someone with an impaired swallow reflex is likely to find clear liquids such as tea or water most difficult to consume.

People should be encouraged to start with easier soft smooth textures such as puréed meat or mashed soft vegetables and progress to a soft diet consistency as their swallow improves.

**TABLE 17 CLASSIFICATION OF MODIFIED THICKNESS AND TEXTURES –
CHALLENGING AND EASIER FOODS**

CHALLENGING FOODS – thickness	EASIER FOODS – thickness
THIN FLUIDS eg water, fruit juice	THICK FLUIDS eg drinking yoghurt, milk shake, thin custard
THIN AND WATERY eg thin yoghurt, thin gravy	THICK AND CREAMY eg creamed potatoes, semolina, ground rice, creamed pulses, thick sauces, thick gravy, thick custard, fromage frais, thick creamy yoghurt
SWIMMING FOODS eg sponge cake swimming in custard, carrots and meat in gravy	
THIN AND LUMPY eg thin rice pudding	THICK AND LUMPY eg meat/fish and vegetables in thick sauces, macaroni cheese, sieved meals.

CHALLENGING FOODS – textures	EASIER FOODS – textures
	SINGLE TEXTURE eg mashed vegetables, mashed banana
CRUNCH AND CRUMBLE OR SPLINTER eg crisp raw apple, raw carrot, crisps, cream crackers, nuts, digestive biscuits	CRUNCH AND DISSOLVE eg cheese puffs, sugar puffs, wafers, sponge fingers
BITE AND STICK eg white bread	BITE AND DISSOLVE eg sponge cake, chocolate buttons
HARD CHEW eg tough meat, dry fish, toffee, chewing gum	SOFT CHEW eg soft raw apple, boiled potato, boiled carrot, processed meat (eg corned beef), brown bread and spread
STRINGY AND HUSKY eg spinach, runner beans, shredded meat, chicken, celery	
BITE AND SLIP eg tinned peaches, oranges, jelly	SOFT SLIP AND SWALLOW eg tinned spaghetti, ice cream, mousse, Angel Delight
TASTE – acid, bitter, savoury	**TASTE** – bland, mild, sweet
TEMPERATURE – very hot/ very cold	**TEMPERATURE** – warm

Depending on the degree of dysphagia the patient may be able to eat:

- a soft diet using minced meat, flaked fish, soft vegetables, mashed potatoes, soft fruit (without skin) and milk puddings, bread (without crusts) and butter, scrambled eggs and omelette;
- a soft and smooth diet using food which is soft and mashed, such as mashed soft vegetables, soft mashed potatoes, thick smooth soup, mashed soft fruit and milk pudding; *or*
- a puréed diet where food is puréed using a blender and additional water added, such as puréed meat, puréed potato, puréed vegetables, smooth yoghurt, mousse and ground rice pudding

As the degree of restriction increases, the likelihood of an inadequate intake intensifies. Also as food is more dilute it can acquire a watery taste and unacceptable appearance. Patients therefore require supplementation to prevent malnutrition (see p 80).

Avoid the following foods:

- mixed textures, such as minestrone soup, oranges
- stringy textures, such as bacon, cabbage, runner beans
- floppy textures, such as lettuce, cucumber
- acidic foods, such as lemons, gooseberries
- food with skins, such as peanuts, peas, sweetcorn, broad beans
- alcohol

As the normal protective cough and gag reflexes are often inhibited, initial feeding must be in a carefully controlled environment with appropriate suction apparatus – and staff trained to use it – available if aspiration is required (see p 113). It takes time, so be patient and bear the following points in mind:

- The client should be seated upright with the head slightly forward so that the neck is not extended and remain in this position for 30 minutes after feeding as a precaution against aspiration.
- The initial food choice should be a smooth, thickened item that has a pleasant appearance such as a smooth yoghurt or blancmange. Only a small quantity should be given as the first goal is to introduce a range of textures to the client. Begin with the textures that are classified as easier foods moving to the more challenging textures later.

- The patient must be made aware of the extent of any reduction in facial or oral sensation. This is particularly true when only one side of the face is affected – you obviously want to avoid the food being retained in the side with the problem.
- General weakness can inhibit the ability to form and manipulate the food bolus in the mouth. Dribbling may occur if lip closure is partial. Exercises are available to develop awareness and control of the lips and face; the Speech and Language Therapist (SALT) – see page 90 – will have details.
- The movements of the tongue and jaw are important for chewing and sucking food. Exercises to strengthen the movement of the tongue and encourage greater jaw control are also available from the SALT.

Menus of possible foods

If someone has severe difficulties with swallowing they may need a purée diet. Table 18 offers a sample 24-hour menu. The person should still be offered a wide variety of food but the consistency may need to change. Remember to:

- Ensure that they eat little and often with snacks between meals, such as milky drinks, yoghurts, commercial meal replacements or prescribed supplements.
- Make the food as nourishing as possible and add extra calories using other foods such as butter or powder supplements (for example Maxijul, Caloreen or Polycal).
- Monitor the nutritional intake very carefully as it may be inadequate and use supplementary products as needed.

CASE STUDY 10

Mr Tom Harold

Mr Harold has had a stroke which has affected his swallowing ability. Lumpy food gets stuck and thin liquids reach the back of his mouth so quickly that he chokes. He therefore requires a purée diet.

> ## Q
> **What foods might you give him?**
> **How would you ensure that he ate enough?**
> **What would Mr Harold need to do when he is eating?**

TABLE 18 SAMPLE 24-HOUR PURÉE DIET

Breakfast	Thickened fruit juice Weetabix soaked in milk or instant breakfast cereal with milk
Mid-morning	Thickened tea/coffee, yoghurt or mousse
Midday	Liquidised casserole/stew Liquidised vegetables (eg carrots) Mashed potato with added butter Thickened custard and purée fruit (eg tinned peaches) in syrup or purée milk pudding (eg ground rice)
Mid-afternoon	Thickened tea/coffee/fruit juice Ice cream and mashed fruit
Evening meal	Thickened soup (with no lumps) Cauliflower cheese (blended) Mashed mushy peas (without skins) Mashed potato with added butter Mashed banana with evaporated milk or thick creamy yoghurt
Bedtime	Milky drink
Snack ideas	Thick natural yoghurt, mousse, fromage frais, Greek yoghurt

Non-oral feeding

Non-oral feeding is used when patients are at risk of aspiration with oral (through the mouth) feeding or are unable to meet their nutritional requirements by that route. Non-oral, or enteral, feeding involves passing a fine bore tube into a part of the digestive tract; the location depends on the medical condition and state of the gut. Types include nasogastric (through the nose), gastrostomy, jejunostomy, nasoduodenal and nasojejunal, depending on the site of insertion of the tube.

Gastrostomy feeding (either G tube or percutaneous endoscopic gastrostomy (PEG) feeding), where the tube is passed directly into the stomach, is often more acceptable for long-term use. The tube does not interfere with oral exercises to stimulate speech, sensation in the facial area or swallow retraining. It also cannot be seen under clothes and therefore may be more acceptable to the patient.

Key decisions in non-oral feeding include:

- Has the regime for an individual patient been decided on a combination of clinical, nutritional and practical grounds? (The medical staff in charge of the patient have the ultimate responsibility.)
- Does the regime over 24 hours meet the energy, fluid and other nutrient needs of the individual?
- Have technical decisions regarding the rate, the maintenance/replacement of the tube and the supply of feed and pump, if needed, been agreed by all concerned?
- Who will administer the feed in a safe hygienic way?
- Are adequate procedures in place to keep accurate records and monitor progress?
- Do staff have sufficient knowledge or is staff training necessary?
- Are the carers able to identify and resolve complications in non-oral feeding?
- Are adequate support mechanisms and referral procedures in place for review?
- Have the wishes of the patient and relatives been considered?
- Does this intervention improve the quality of life for the patient?

Complications of nasogastric feeding

Many patients experience some discomfort with non-oral feeding but the number of complications can be reduced with good hygiene practices and careful administration of the feed. Nasogostric (through the nose) feeding is the most frequently used method of non-oral feeding. The most common problems are identified with their potential consequences in Table 19.

TABLE 19 COMMON PROBLEMS WITH NASOGASTRIC FEEDING

Problem	Potential consequence
Medication given through tube Tube not flushed regularly	Tube blocked
Patient coughing Tube irritating nose	Tube pulled out or displaced
Medication including antibiotics Rapid infusion rate Bacterial contamination of feed	Diarrhoea
Improper patient position Medication Rapid infusion rate	Nausea and vomiting
Wrong quantity of fluids (total volume including intravenous)	Dehydration or over-hydration
Wrong patient position (patient should not be horizontal but fed with their head and shoulders raised).	Choking, aspiration

Strict hygiene practices should be observed when tube feeding is used.

If you are involved in tube feeding you should have the support and advice of the district nurse and specialist nurse and dietitian. Most of the companies that produce feeding tubes also have a telephone advisory service and specialist technical advisers who will provide additional support and training.

8 Nutrition and Dementia

This chapter examines the particular needs of older people with dementia. It discusses nutrition-related problems and also suggests some strategies to assist food intake, including the role of finger foods.

Prevalence and signs and symptoms

It is estimated that 40 per cent of older people suffer from mental illness. Ten per cent have organic changes in the brain resulting in acute confusional state or dementia. The remaining 30 per cent are affected functionally with no biological brain changes. They may be anxious, paranoid or depressed. These symptoms are often triggered by changes in circumstances such as bereavement of a partner or another loss, whether of status, income, health, company, independence or mobility for example.

Dementia is an irreversible impairment of the higher cerebral functions which affects social behaviour, emotional control, visual-motor skills, recognition of complex relationships, and the ability to learn tasks and to remember recent events.

Alzheimer's disease is the most common form of dementia in older people and affects about 20 per cent of people over 75 years. The individual experiences progressive (initially short-term) loss of intellectual ability and memory. Eventually they become unable to recognise near relatives. The second most common cause of irreversible dementia is multi-infarct dementia which is a result of many small strokes in the brain. A further 10 per cent of dementia cases may be the result of such conditions as alcoholism, depression, cerebral tumours, thyroid disease and vitamin B12 deficiency.

The medical treatment of all cases of mental illness must be considered carefully and the cause or causes investigated and if possible resolved. Acute confusional state (ACS) can often be treated provided the cause is identified, which might be for example dehydration or drug side effects.

Mental illness may lead to many changes in food intake, perhaps most strikingly in depressive illnesses, where apathy and loss of appetite (anorexia) may further influence the diet. In these cases it is important to treat the depression, either by medication or counselling, and to consider the impact, if any, on nutritional status and more importantly on the client's nutritional intake. Weight loss and changes in specific behaviour related to food should be recorded in the medical examination. As a secondary feature of depression, there is often a diminished interest and pleasure in most activities and consequently it is very likely that individuals will reduce their interest in food and cooking.

Alzheimer's disease is a progressive disorder which can be divided into three stages. In the first stage there is loss of memory, partial disorientation and lack of spontaneous emotional response. The second stage is characterised by an inability to identify familiar sights, sounds or smells. The person may not recognise family members or familiar settings, food or eating utensils. Erratic non-purposeful movements may begin at this stage. In the third stage seizures develop, speech is lost and patients are indifferent to their environment. Non-purposeful movements may become more intense. Sufferers usually have little interest in food or food is often played with rather than eaten. As the disease progresses to the final stage, patients might show signs of compulsive eating or alternatively refuse to eat or try to eat objects that are inedible.

Age Concern Books publishes *The Dementia Care Training Pack* (see p 126) which covers general topics related to caring for older people with dementia. The Alzheimer's Disease Society (address on p 121) can offer information and advice.

TABLE 20 SIGNS AND SYMPTOMS OF DEMENTIA AND POSSIBLE GENERAL CONSEQUENCES

Signs and symptoms	Possible general consequences
Impaired memory	early – little confused and forgetful, memory becomes less reliable late – progressive failure of memory and decline in ability to think clearly independent living increasingly hazardous
Disorientation	loses all track of time (eg going back in time or going to bed fully dressed) denial/lack of awareness of location (eg getting lost in familiar surroundings or unable to recall own house) failure to recognise close relatives
Lack of judgement	inappropriate expenditure of money refusal to pay bills failure to collect pension or going daily for pension failure to observe proper precautions in traffic
Loss of emotional control	blunting of emotions with an apparent disregard for the feelings of others aggressive outbursts frustrated, irritable and angry when cannot remember
Personality and interpersonal relations	temper groundless accusations rejection of attentions
Miscellaneous offensive behaviours	restless wandering by day indoors knocking at neighbours' door pilfering denial of misbehaviour
Delusions and hallucinations	due to poor recent memory and sensory impairment (vision or hearing) paranoia hearing voices and/or seeing things that do not exist

Memory loss is often one of the most disturbing symptoms for the individual and carers (Table 21). It can bring about a marked impact in food and fluid intake. Monitoring should be carried out so that an accurate estimate is obtained of the food and fluid consumed.

TABLE 21 POSSIBLE OUTCOMES OF MEMORY LOSS

Issue	Possible result
Talk/conversation	early – does not admit shortcomings, leading to inappropriate conversations, perhaps betraying confidence unintentionally speech – slurred, aphasia repetitive questioning
Impairment of domestic skills	insufficient/excessive food purchased forgets to buy food failure to prepare meals food allowed to go stale but still eaten inappropriate material consumed gas left on kettle, pots and pans burnt out failure to complete task accumulation of rubbish refuses food
Lapses in dressing and feeding	habits and skills acquired over a lifetime seem to be abandoned forgets order in which clothes are worn inappropriate choice of dress failure to fasten clothing stripping all clothing objectionable eating of food
Lapses in personal hygiene	refusal to bath or wash failure to close door while using the toilet urination in places other than the toilet (not due to incontinence) offensive odour

Nutrition-related consequences

Many of the signs and symptoms of dementia can impact on nutrition. Nutrition-related problems differ in the different stages of the disease (Table 22). In the early phase there will be such things as forgetting to eat, eating food which is too hot, eating non-foods, gorging, eating spoilt foods, and difficulties in relation to shopping, cooking and storing food. There is often a change in food choice, sometimes in terms of a preference for sweet and salty foods and sometimes unusual food choices, for example eating a jar of mayonnaise. Some people may also have physical problems that occur concurrently, which interfere with their mobility and have an impact on their feeding ability and possibly also on their ability to co-ordinate chewing, swallowing and facial movements.

TABLE 22 NUTRITION-RELATED CONSEQUENCES OF DEMENTIA

Sign and symptoms	Example of nutrition consequence
Impaired memory	early – forgets to put milk in tea late – may not turn gas cooker off, lets saucepan boil dry and does not notice cannot remember if eaten or not
Disorientation	eats breakfast at lunchtime does not recognise own kitchen
Lack of judgement	purchases large quantities of a food item unnecessarily inappropriate portion sizes failure to recognise when food is spoilt
Loss of emotional control	rejects food prepared by spouse suddenly and aggressively decides will not eat a familiar food
Personality and interpersonal relations	accuses people of stealing food rejects efforts of others to help
Miscellaneous offensive behaviours	takes food off other people's plates objectionable eating of food may eat non-food items
Delusions and hallucinations	'hears voices' telling them to eat or not eat a particular food

During the second phase there is an increase in activity with the patient becoming agitated. There may be increased appetite but often still an inadequate intake. Food can be hoarded in the mouth rather than swallowed and the ability to use cutlery properly is diminished.

In the final phase food is often not recognised and patients may refuse to open their mouths or turn away when food is offered. The patient is unable to ask for food or drink and may have difficulty swallowing and initiating movements to open their mouth or chew. It can be very difficult for patients and carers as the disease progresses and support mechanisms should be available for staff.

Weight loss in dementia

Weight loss is common in patients with dementia. Table 23 identifies some reasons and suggests interventions. The most common reason is a reduced food intake due to physical difficulties in eating or memory impairment. Studies have shown that it is important to monitor the food eaten rather than that offered.

The overall aim is to help a person to retain their independence. Therefore it is important to remember that:

- An individual's ability to feed themselves will remain longer than good table manners.
- Malnutrition can cause further mental impairment.

Try to maintain an encouraging, friendly atmosphere and positive approach to mealtimes. A relaxed atmosphere with minimal distractions may help to improve the food intake. Points to bear in mind include:

- Minimise distractions (such as the television) at mealtimes.
- Take into account that some individuals eat better alone than in groups.
- Do not fill glasses and cups to the top but allow room for shaking as a person moves the glass or cup to their mouth.
- Present only one course at a time.
- If the person has difficulty using normal utensils, modified ones

should have been selected with the help of the occupational therapist.

■ Have essential items only on the table. Condiments should be offered then removed.

■ Plan the menu to suit the person's level of eating skill (they may need bite size chunks for example).

■ Ensure that portion sizes are appropriate to the individual.

■ Avoid mixed textures of foods.

■ Ensure food is served at the correct temperature and that hot food for example is not too hot.

TABLE 23 WEIGHT LOSS IN DEMENTIA: POTENTIAL INTERVENTIONS

Possible reason for weight loss	Potential nutritional assessment and intervention
Low food intake	monitor food intake adequate supervision of eating assess swallowing and chewing ability are dentures fitting properly?
Other health problems	check for other illnesses
Increased energy expenditure	is patient agitated, hungry or dehydrated? assess activity level
Malabsorption	stool examination
Increased metabolism	assess energy requirements
Drug interactions	review medications
Nutritional deficiency	review food intake

Finger foods

Finger foods can be held easily while eating and can be eaten without cutlery and at room temperature. When people have difficulty handling cutlery, finger foods are a means of maintaining independence. This way of presenting food is also helpful for other individuals who eat slowly or have a limited attention span.

Table 24 provides some examples. Some individuals may find some of these items too dry to swallow, in which case moist finger foods should be encouraged.

TABLE 24 EXAMPLES OF FINGER FOODS

Bread and cereals	Vegetables
Biscuits	Broccoli spears – cooked
Buttered toast fingers	Carrot sticks
Cereal bar	Chips
Chapattis	New potatoes
Crackers with butter	Fried plantain
Fruit loaf	Sliced cucumber
Prawn crackers	Quartered tomatoes
Sandwiches	Bhajies

Meat, fish, cheese	Fruit
Sliced meat	Apples – sliced
Sausages	Banana
Meatballs	Grapes
Pizza	Mandarin orange segments
Pork pie – slice	
Quiche	
Fish fingers	
Cheese on toast	
Cheese cubes	
Hard-boiled eggs	
Kebabs	
Chicken pieces	

Snacks
Ice cream cone
Dried apricots
Marmite on toast

(Source: VOICES 1998)

Further information is available in *Eating Well for Older People with Dementia*, a publication from Voluntary Organisations Involved in Caring in the Elderly Sector (VOICES). Copies are available from Eating Well for Older People with Dementia, PO Box 5, Manchester M60 3GE, price £12.99.

CASE STUDY 11

Miss Vera Lawrence

Miss Lawrence is 82 years old and physically mobile. Her short-term memory is gradually deteriorating so that she cannot remember what she has eaten and even whether she has had a meal.

She tends to eat a small amount of food and then leave the table as she is unable to sit still for a meal. She becomes agitated if forced to remain seated.

Q What short-term measures might you suggest to ensure that Miss Lawrence eats and drinks enough?
How might you monitor the situation?
In the longer term, as Miss Lawrence's dementia worsens, what practical support is she likely to require at mealtimes?

CASE STUDIES – SOME SUGGESTED ANSWERS

Case study 1 – Mrs Elizabeth Jones

Did you consider why she was not eating? Possible reasons might include her reaction to living in an institution – new resident, lonely, strange environment, loss of freedom, meals at a different time, unfamiliar food, eating with others, missing a pet or neighbour.

Find out about her previous lifestyle prior to admission – how active was she and did she have friends and relatives who visited and perhaps cannot now as the home is not as accessible?

Find out about her previous eating habits – appetite, likes and dislikes. Was her admission planned or due to a sudden problem? Many people experience problems in adjusting to institutional living.

Consider favourite foods, small meals, preferred seating arrangement, introducing her to other residents and ensuring that she feels valued and accepted. Many of these points are covered in detail in Chapter 4.

Case study 2 – Mr Mohammed Aftab

His religious and cultural needs must be considered. Religious needs include types of food, cooking methods and meal service. Food should be halal. Family members and the local religious leader could be consulted.

Washing and prayer facilities will be needed and a separate lounge and eating areas for men and women may be required.

Did you consider how much he might have adapted his diet to Western foods? Many people from Pakistan have maintained their traditional food habits. Do you have access to a suitable cook who could explain and demonstrate how to prepare curries and other food items correctly?

Case study 3 – Mrs Hilda Hulse

Ask Mrs Hulse about her eating habits prior to admission; she may be used to having a larger meal in the evening. Take steps to ensure that she does not feel threatened and that she will not be labelled a difficult resident.

Talk to her daughter about her complaint. The problem may relate to type and timing of meals rather than the quantity served.

Mrs Hulse should be offered an evening snack such as a milky drink and cheese and crackers – ask what food items she would prefer.

This is an opportunity to find out if other residents are hungry in the evening. Is the evening meal served too early and the bedtime snack inadequate?

Case study 4 – Miss Alison Sutherland

Reasons why Miss Sutherland does not finish her drinks may include:

- fear about not being able to get to the toilet in time
- not feeling thirsty
- the hot drink goes cold
- drink not to her taste (for example tea is too strong)
- on 'water tablets' (diuretics).

Ask about her preferred drinks.

Some routine help should be available to reach the toilet so that Miss Sutherland does not feel she has to ask or is pressurised.

Explain why it is important to drink eight to ten cups of liquid a day.

Check her medication for possible side reactions.

Explain that 'water tablets' do not mean that you have to drink less liquid.

Constipation is often due to a lack of fluid and fibre in the diet. Encourage Miss Sutherland to eat more fibre rich foods (see pp 51–52). Eating wholegrain breakfast cereal and using wholemeal bread could be easy changes.

Why does she have difficulty eating fruit – does she have problems with her teeth and chewing or difficulties peeling an orange? Perhaps the fruit could be prepared for Miss Sutherland or a dental check might be needed?

Case study 5 – Miss Lily Bushell

Ask Miss Bushell if she has any difficulty eating any particular food items. It may be that her dentures or natural teeth need attention and that she cannot chew meat properly and has therefore avoided red meat. If so, arrange for a dentist to visit.

Which food items did you decide were rich in iron? Encourage Miss Bushell to eat the iron rich foods that she enjoys (see p 55). Consult Miss Bushell in this process, initially by asking her likes and dislikes. Eating vitamin C rich foods (such as fruit) with iron foods aids absorption. If Miss Bushell is consuming a large quantity of strong tea with her meals, this may inhibit iron absorption.

Case study 6 – Mrs Freda Baxter

If Mrs Baxter lost some weight by reducing the amount of sugar and sugary foods eaten, she would feel better and her diabetes would be controlled.

Explain that her dry mouth is likely to be due to the poorly controlled diabetes. Non-energy alternatives should be used instead of the boiled sweets.

Obvious sources of highly concentrated sugar should be eliminated, such as sugar in tea and other sweetened drinks such as squashes and fizzy pop. Non-energy artificial sweeteners can have a role, particularly for the overweight patient.

'Diabetic products' are unnecessary and in many cases contain a similar amount of dietary energy to their equivalent normal food item although they may be much more expensive. Perhaps her daughter could provide treats which are not food items or bring low calorie sugar-free drinks and fruit.

Mrs Baxter needs to eat regularly throughout the day but reduce the quantity consumed so that she achieves a slow steady weight loss of about 2 kilograms a month.

Swap her sweet sherry to a dry sherry, reduce the quantity or offer her an alternative spirit drink with a sugar-free mixer.

Case study 7 – Mrs Anila Khan

Check that these are her own clothes.

Ask Mrs Khan if she thinks that she has lost weight, then weigh her and compare to previous weights. Any weight change should be noted and the reason determined.

Weight change is often the first sign of an illness. An unintentional weight change of 3 kilograms in three months should be investigated. Have you got a policy to ensure that this occurs and adequate equipment which is regularly checked? Residents who are more vulnerable should be weighed more often and appropriate interventions started if any unintentional weight loss occurs.

Case study 8 – Mr John Godfrey

Consider the environment – is it pleasant and relaxed with sufficient time to eat without distractions or offensive smells? Mr Godfrey needs to be seated comfortably in an upright position, supported where necessary, with the table at a suitable height.

The food needs to be tasty and served at the correct temperature to encourage someone to eat. A small glass of sherry, brandy or beer before a meal can help to stimulate the appetite (provided it is medically acceptable).

Offer small quantities of food at frequent intervals throughout the day and evening (see pp 80–81).

Increase the nutrient value by adding other food items which do not increase the bulk of the original food (such as butter or margarine added to potatoes). Use fortified milk in place of ordinary milk throughout the day (see p 81). Supplementary products may be useful in the short term while Mr Godfrey regains his appetite but normal food should be encouraged.

Case study 9 – Mrs Irene Morgan

As eating and drinking may be a laborious process requiring assistance, people who have had a stroke may have an inadequate energy and nutrient intake. Consequently an individual may lose weight and can become malnourished. Many people experience some difficulty with one or more aspects of eating following their stroke. Problems might include:

■ Reduced ability to communicate – Mrs Morgan cannot express herself verbally and will therefore experience some frustration. A code system could be developed with a set of pictures to point at for example.

■ Reduced concentration – the attention span is reduced so that she may be easily distracted from the task in hand.

■ Restricted hand/arm movement and limited strength – Mrs Morgan has partial paralysis of her arm and will be unable to lift or grip cutlery or food items with her left hand. Cutlery with a wide and/or soft handle may be helpful for her right hand.

■ Reduced hand to mouth co-ordination – can Mrs Morgan lift the food from the plate to the mouth or is she 'missing her mouth'?

■ Eating – is Mrs Morgan experiencing a reduced ability to chew certain foods, incomplete lip closure with dribbling or an inability to manipulate the tongue? A reduced facial sensation in one side of the mouth may mean that food is pouched.

■ Dry mouth – lack of saliva production may mean that Mrs Morgan cannot form a bolus with her food.

Did you think about issues such as: seating, cutlery, special aids, what help is required with eating and what types of food are most appropriate (cut the meat for example)?

You will need to monitor any weight changes and intervene if Mrs Morgan is losing weight.

Case study 10 – Mr Tom Harold

A puréed diet is where food is puréed using a blender and additional water added. The initial food choice should be a smooth thickened item that has a pleasant appearance such as a smooth yoghurt or thickened custard.

Keep a food and fluid chart to record what has been offered and consumed. As the degree of restriction increases, the likelihood of an inadequate intake intensifies. Also as food is more dilute it can acquire a watery taste and unacceptable appearance. Patients therefore require supplementation to prevent malnutrition.

Mr Harold should be seated upright with the head slightly forward so that his neck is not extended and he should remain in this position for 30 minutes after feeding as a precaution against aspiration.

Mr Harold must be made aware of the extent of any reduction in facial or oral sensation. General weakness can inhibit the ability to form and manipulate the food bolus in the mouth. Dribbling may occur if lip closure is partial.

Case study 11 – Miss Vera Lawrence

Think about Miss Lawrence's seating position, including where she sits in relation to the other residents. Offer verbal prompts to encourage eating and small frequent meals. Consider the use of finger foods and a suitable bag to carry then. Ask about and record her favourite foods, likes and dislikes, offering some of her favourites as appropriate.

Miss Lawrence is likely to be aware of her loss of memory and may be distressed. Her longer-term memory may be intact. Talk respectfully about the past.

You will need to monitor food intake and wastage and also monitor her weight and weight change to ensure that she is getting sufficient food energy.

In the longer term as her physical ability deteriorates, remember that being neat and tidy is not the most important factor – self-feeding, even if a bit messy, should be encouraged.

Assistance with feeding and drinking will be required. It is helpful if it is generally the same people who remain with her for the whole meal. Some people lose the ability to use a knife and fork and may prefer a spoon, but later will need feeding.

Cut meat and offer food at appropriate texture and temperature and in appropriate quantities – smaller servings may be helpful.

Did you consider the potential difficulties with oral behaviour? These can include difficulty with chewing, holding food in the mouth, forgetting to chew or swallow, biting the spoon or refusing to open the mouth. Individual strategies might include providing easier food, offering verbal cues, gentle massage of the cheek or using a plastic spoon.

Did you remember to think about what kinds of support the staff might need as well?

GLOSSARY

Ageing process Normal physiological and biochemical changes that occur in the body with age.

Anaemia A disease characterised by a deficiency of blood as a whole or of haemoglobin in the blood. Iron and/or folate deficiency are the most common forms of nutritional anaemia.

Aphasia Loss of the power of remembering words and expressing ideas in words, often as the result of a brain disease.

Aspartame An artificial sweetener that does not contain any energy (calories) and can therefore be used by an overweight person to sweeten drinks if needed.

Aspiration The removal of fluids from a cavity in the body by suction. When someone has difficulty swallowing, food and fluid may get into the lung instead of passing down the oesophagus into the stomach. Normally if food and fluid enters the airway the cough reflex starts. With swallowing difficulties, the food stays in the lungs and can cause illness. Aspiration is the act of withdrawing the food that has 'gone the wrong way'.

Astigmatism A defect of the eye linked with dimness of vision due to a malformation of the lens of the eye.

Bolus A round mass. In the mouth food is chewed and mixed with saliva to form a bolus which is then swallowed.

BMI (Body Mass Index) A figure used to demonstrate the relationship in an individual between height and body weight. Using standard charts the figure can be used to give an indication of health – whether you are average weight, underweight or overweight for your height.

Community meal A meal provided to an older person or other vulnerable individual in the community. It may be delivered already cooked or frozen to the person's house or served to them at a lunch club.

Decalcification Removal of calcium from the bone.

Demispan A physical measure which can be used instead of height. It is the distance from the web of the fingers (between the middle and ring fingers) and the sternal notch when the subject's arm is horizontal to their side and is usually measured with a steel tape. Demispan does not appear to be affected by the ageing process, unlike height which is reduced.

Dextrin A soluble carbohydrate. Not as sweet as sugar.

Diabetes Common chronic disorder where the body cannot secrete insulin from the pancreas in sufficient quantities to absorb the food eaten. The person with diabetes has a raised blood glucose unless treated.

Diuretics Drugs that stimulate the production of urine. They are used in a range of medical conditions, for example heart failure, where the body is retaining too much water in the cells.

Diverticula A series of pouch-like projections along the lining (or wall) of the large bowel. Food waste can get stuck in these pouches and sometimes they become inflamed. This is called diverticulitis and can be painful and cause diarrhoea.

DRV Dietary Reference Value. A term used to cover LRNI, EAR, RNI and Safe Intake. It indicates the nutritional requirements for groups of healthy people.

Dysphagia A medical term for difficulty in swallowing.

EAR Estimated Average Requirements of a group of people for energy or protein or a vitamin or mineral. About half will usually need more than the EAR and half less.

Enteral feed When someone is fed via a fine tube either through the nose into the gut or directly into a specific part of the gut. The feed in liquid form is balanced and therefore can sustain someone nutritionally.

Folate or folic acid A water soluble vitamin that is destroyed during long cooking. Rich sources are liver, yeast and dark green vegetables. A deficiency causes a common form of anaemia.

Fructose A type of sugar naturally occurring in fruits.

Halal meat Meat that is killed according to Islamic food laws.

Homeostatic regulation Mechanisms within the body to maintain itself. These are less efficient in older people meaning that older people are more susceptible to sudden changes in temperature – in a cold situation they start shivering later and in response to heat sweat later. Hypothermia or overheating and dehydration are thus more common.

Hyperlipidaemia A medical condition where too much fat is circulating in the blood. The excess fat is likely to be deposited on the wall lining of the blood vessels, restricting the passage of blood.

Hypoglycaemic drugs A range of drugs used in the treatment of diabetes. Sometimes known as hypoglycaemic agents (OHA).

Hypothyroidism A condition that occurs when the thyroid gland is underactive. Once it has been diagnosed, drug intervention is usually effective.

Insulin A hormone secreted by the pancreas which is essential for the absorption of carbohydrates. People with diabetes do not secrete sufficient insulin and may therefore require artificial supplies injected at regular intervals.

Intrinsic sugars Sugars that are part of the natural food structure.

kJ Kilojoule = 1,000 joules. A unit used to measure the energy value of food.

Kosher/Koshering Food that has been slaughtered according to Jewish food regulations.

Lean body mass The body is made up of water, fat, bone and lean body mass. Lean body mass is the muscles and organs. The amount of lean body mass can decline with ageing, for example because of lack of activity and subsequent muscle wasting.

Life expectancy How many years a person is expected to live.

Life span Maximum number of years people can live. Currently this is considered to between 110 and 120 years.

LRNI Lower Reference Nutrient Intake for protein or a vitamin or mineral. An amount of the nutrient that is enough for only the few people in a society who have low needs.

Malnutrition ('Poor nutrition') This occurs when the food consumed is not able to match the physiological and other nutrient requirements in the body. The person usually loses weight and becomes deficient in particular nutrients. When someone is malnourished they take longer to recover after an illness.

Maltose A sugar similar in structure to table sugar (sucrose) but not as sweet and which occurs naturally in the brewing process.

Microgram (μg) One-millionth of 1 gram.

Milligram (mg) One-thousandth of 1 gram.

MJ Megajoule = 1 million joules.

Multi-infarct dementia Dementia that has developed as a result of a series of small strokes in the brain.

Non-milk extrinsic sugars (NMES) Obvious sugars outside the normal food structure. The most common is table sugar (sucrose).

Non-starch polysaccharides (NSP) Sometimes called dietary fibre. As a population we are encouraged to eat more.

Nutritional assessment An assessment of the nutritional status of someone. It may consist of assessing the current and previous food intake, appetite, body weight and social and medical conditions related to food.

Nutritional intake The amount of food and fluid consumed expressed in terms of nutrients (eg protein, vitamin C) rather than as food (eg potatoes).

Nutritional requirements For any nutrient this is the amount of that nutrient needed by the individual, usually expressed for a group of healthy individuals with similar characteristics such as age and sex. Nutritional requirements can be increased in illness, particularly fever or trauma.

Nutritional status The current state of an individual in terms of nutrition.

Obesity Is said to occur when an individual's BMI is greater than 30 – ie they are too heavy for their height and would achieve a health benefit from losing weight.

Oedema Excess fluid in the tissues of the body.

Packed cell volume (PCV) A haematological measure of the volume of cells in the blood. When reduced it can be an indicator of anaemia.

Peripheral nerve sensitivity The nerves in the fingers can become less sensitive with ageing and because of some chronic diseases.

Phytate Phytic acid, present in some cereals, inhibits the absorption of certain minerals (such as copper and iron) in the bowel by converting the copper (ferrous) and iron (ferric) salts into insoluble phytates.

Polyunsaturated fat Fats can be divided into saturated, monounsaturated and polyunsaturated, depending on their structure. Polyunsaturated fats are believed to be more beneficial; but as a population we need to reduce the total fat consumed.

Prescribed supplement A supplementary product given under medical direction. May be in liquid, powder or dessert form.

Retinol Pre-formed vitamin A – from animal sources – which can be stored in the body. When these stores are depleted the mucus lining is affected and resistance to infection is reduced. In the eye the result of this is called 'night blindness' but if not treated it can lead to more severe changes and eventual blindness. The mucus lining in the gut and lungs are also affected meaning that the individual is more susceptible to gut disturbances such as diarrhoea and respiratory tract infections.

Riboflavin One of the B group of vitamins. It is destroyed by sunlight. Important food sources are milk, eggs, liver, meat and fish. A deficiency may lead to cracked lips, sores at the corner of the mouth and a rough skin.

RNI Reference Nutrient Intake for protein or a vitamin or a mineral. An amount of the nutrient that is enough, or more than enough, for about 97 per cent of people in a group. If the average intake of a group is at the RNI, then the risk of deficiency in the group is very small.

Safe Intake A term used to indicate intake or a range of intakes of a nutrient for which there is not enough information to estimate RNI, EAR or LRNI. It is an amount that is enough for almost everyone but not so large as to cause undesirable effects.

Thiamin One of the B group of vitamins. This vitamin is needed for the absorption of carbohydrates and so more is needed when a person consumes such a diet. Meat, poultry and fish are rich sources and wholegrain cereals contain a useful supply. The clinical deficiency (beriberi) is rare in the UK but may occur among people with chronic high alcohol intakes.

Triglyceride Food fats consist of a mixture of triglycerides. Each triglyceride consists of three fatty acids with a unit of glycerol. The differences between one fat or oil and another are largely the result of the different fatty acids in each.

REFERENCES AND FURTHER READING

Biggs, J 1997. *The Catering Checklist*. Trowbridge: The Advisory Body for Social Services Catering.

Bond, S 1997. *Eating Matters: A resource for improving dietary care in hospitals*. Newcastle: University of Newcastle Centre for Health Service Research.

British Diabetic Association; Nutrition Subcommittee 1991. 'Dietary recommendations for people with diabetes: an update for the 1990s'. *Journal of Human Nutrition and Diatetics*, 4, pp 393-412.

British Dietetic Association; Nutrition Advisory Group for Elderly People 1996. *In the Minority through the 90's: A handbook for those who provide meals for elderly people in a multicultural society*. Leeds: Nutrition Advisory Group for Elderly People (NAGE) – see page 120.

British Medical Journal editorial 1997. 'Aging: a subject that must be at the top of the world agendas'. *BMJ*, 315, pp 1029-1030.

Davies, L and Holdsworth, D 1979. 'A–Z checklist: a technique for assessing nutritional 'at risk' factors in residential homes for the elderly'. *Journal of Human Nutrition*, 33, pp 165-169.

Department of Health (DoH) 1991. *Dietary Reference Values for Food Energy and Nutrients for the United Kingdom*. (Report of the Committee on Medical Aspects of Food Policy No 41.) London: HMSO.

Department of Health (DoH) 1992. *The Nutrition of Elderly People*. (Report of the Committee on Medical Aspects of Food Policy No 43.) London: HMSO.

Finch, S et al 1998. *National Diet and Nutrition Survey: People aged 65 years and over. Volume 1*. London: The Stationery Office (TSO).

Health Advisory Service 2000 (HAS) 1998. *Not Because They are Old*. London: HAS.

Health Education Authority (HEA) 1994. *The Balance of Good Health*. London: HEA/DoH.

Maslow, AH 1943. 'A theory of human motivation'. *Psychological Reviews*, *50*, pp 370-396.

McWhirter, JP and Pennington, CR 1994. 'Incidence and recognition of malnutrition in hospital'. *British Medical Journal*, *308*, pp 945-948.

Nutrition Task Force (NTF) 1994. *Eat Well*. London: Department of Health (DoH).

Nutrition Task Force (NTF) 1995. *Eat Well for Older People*. London: DoH.

Nutrition Task Force (NTF) 1996. *Eat Well ii: progress report*. London: DoH.

Steele, JG et al 1998. *National Diet and Nutrition Survey: People aged 65 years and over. Volume 2*. London: TSO.

Caroline Walker Trust 1995. *Eating Well for Older People: Practical and nutritional guidelines for food in residential and nursing homes and for community meals*. London: Caroline Walker Trust.

Caroline Walker Trust 1998. *Catering for Older People in Residential Accommodation (CORA): Menu planner*. London: Caroline Walker Trust.

Voluntary Organisations Involved in Caring in the Elderly Sector (VOICES) 1988. *Eating Well for Older People with Dementia*. Manchester: VOICES.

Webb, G 1995. *Nutrition: A health promotion approach*. London: Arnold.

Webb, G and Copeman, JP 1996. *The Nutrition of Older Adults*. London: Arnold with Age Concern.

World Health Organisation (WHO) 1998. *Population Ageing: A public health challenge* (WHO fact sheet). Geneva: WHO.

Other titles produced by the Nutrition Advisory Group for Elderly People (NAGE) of the British Dietetic Association include:

Eating Through the 90s – this booklet provides information on nutrition and dietetics for those involved in catering for any group of older people.

Fibre Keeps you Fit – this 10 minute video discusses constipation and makes suggestions as to how carers and older people can reduce the incidence of constipation.

Nutrition Assessment Checklist and Guidance Notes – a screening tool for use by health professionals when interviewing older people.

Stimulating a Small Appetite – a 14 minute video, giving practical suggestions, including enriching food and using supplements.

Supermarket Shopping and the Store Cupboard – each sequence in this training video lasts ten minutes and is intended to stimulate discussion.

Taking Steps to Tackle Eating Problems – a handbook and poster for those who care for older people.

Available from NAGE, The British Dietetic Association, Unit 21 Goldthorpe Industrial Estate, Goldthorpe, Rotherham, South Yorkshire S63 9BL. Please send an sae for an order form.

USEFUL ADDRESSES

Alzheimer's Disease Society
Gordon House
10 Greencoat Place
London SW1P 1PH
Tel: 020 7306 0606

Information, support and advice about caring for someone with Alzheimer's disease. Can also direct you to regional and local groups.

British Diabetic Association
10 Queen Anne Street
London W1M 0BD
Tel: 020 7323 1531
Careline: 020 7636 6112

Provides help and support to people diagnosed with diabetes, their families and those who care for them.

Carers National Association
20-25 Glasshouse Yard
London EC1A 4JS
Tel: 020 7490 8818

Provides information and advice if you are looking after someone, whether in your own home or at a distance. Can put you in touch with other carers and carers' groups in your area.

Disabled Living Foundation
380–384 Harrow Road
London W9 2HU
Tel: 020 7289 6111

Information about aids and equipment to help cope with a disability.

Parkinson's Disease Society
215 Vauxhall Bridge Road
London SW1V 1EJ
Tel: 020 7931 8080

Support and information for relatives and carers of someone with Parkinson's disease.

Royal Institute of Public Health and Hygiene (RIPHH)
28 Portland Place
London W1N 4DE
Tel: 020 7580 2731

Runs training courses related to nutrition.

The Stroke Association
CHSA House
123–127 Whitecross Street
London EC1Y 8JJ
Tel: 020 7490 7999

Information and advice if you are caring for someone who has had a stroke.

ABOUT AGE CONCERN

Nutritional Care for Older People: A guide to good practice is one of a wide range of publications produced by Age Concern England, the National Council on Ageing. Age Concern cares about all older people and believes later life should be fulfilling and enjoyable. For too many this is impossible. As the leading charitable movement in the UK concerned with ageing and older people, Age Concern finds effective ways to change that situation.

Where possible, we enable older people to solve problems themselves, providing as much or as little support as they need. Our network of 1,400 local groups, supported by 250,000 volunteers, provides community-based services such as lunch clubs, day centres and home visiting.

Nationally, we take a lead role in campaigning, parliamentary work, policy analysis, research, specialist information and advice provision, and publishing. Innovative programmes promote healthier lifestyles and provide older people with opportunities to give the experience of a lifetime back to their communities.

Age Concern is dependent on donations, covenants and legacies.

Age Concern England
1268 London Road
London SW16 4ER
Tel: 020 8765 7200
Fax: 020 8765 7211

Age Concern Scotland
113 Rose Street
Edinburgh EH2 3DT
Tel: 0131 220 3345
Fax: 0131 220 2779

Age Concern Cymru
4th Floor
1 Cathedral Road
Cardiff CF1 9SD
Tel: 029 2037 1566
Fax: 029 2039 9562

Age Concern Northern Ireland
3 Lower Crescent
Belfast BT7 1NR
Tel: 028 9024 5729
Fax: 028 9023 5497

PUBLICATIONS FROM AGE CONCERN BOOKS

HEALTH & CARE

Know Your Medicines

Pat Blair

The new edition of this handy guide explains many of the common questions older people – and those who care for them – may have about the medicines they use and how this may affect them. Topics covered include:

- what medicines actually do
- using medicines more effectively
- getting advice and asking questions
- taking medicines safely
- medicines and the body system
- common ailments

Other areas covered include advice on dose and strength, different brands, storage and disposal, living in a residential home and an index to look up medicines prescribed. Informative and comprehensive, this new edition is a valuable source of advice and guidance.

£7.99   0-86242-226-4

Caring for Someone with Diabetes

Marina Lewycka

This book brings you up-to-date information about diabetes and how you can live with this condition. Packed with practical help and guidance, this book explores topics such as:

- understanding diabetes
- day to day care
- healthy eating and living
- medication and coping with emergencies

Always positive and supportive, it draws on the experience of people with diabetes and their carers to tell you what you can expect and contains a wealth of useful contact details.

£6.99   0-86242-282-5

Caring for Someone with an Alcohol Problem

Mike Ward

Caring for someone with an alcohol problem can be physically and emotionally exhausting, and it is often difficult to think about what can be done to make things easier. Supportive, positive and full of valuable information, this book offers advice on how to cope as well as comprehensive guidance on steps that can be taken to help the situation.

£6.99   0-86242-227-2

BOOKS FOR PROFESSIONALS WORKING WITH OLDER PEOPLE

Business Skills for Care Management: A guide to costing, contracting and negotiating

Penny Mares

Buying care services for users is now part of everyday practice for many care managers, social workers and other health and care professionals. This book provides the practical, administrative and financial skills that are needed to do the job well. Always practical and accessible, this easy to read book guides the reader through all the key stages involved, emphasising throughout that the aim is to achieve the best quality service for users.

£11.99   0-86242-191-8

Residents' Money: A guide to good practice in care homes

This guide is for people who work in residential and nursing homes who may be involved in handling residents' money or in helping them to manage their financial affairs. It includes detailed advice for care managers and staff on how to design and implement policies that reflect the best in good practice.

£7.99   0-86242-205-1

The Dementia Care Training Pack

Suzette Ansell

This Training Pack is designed for use by managers, proprietors, qualified nurses, and senior carers in residential care settings, the community and hospitals. It addresses the most important areas related to understanding and caring for older people with dementia. Designed in six units – which can be used separately – this training pack aims to facilitate the teaching of junior staff, care assistants and community carers in a variety of situations. The individual units cover:

- dementia – what is it?
- assessing and planning daily needs
- understanding incontinence
- communication
- challenging and disruptive behaviour
- drug therapy

The pack contains: 27 key point overhead transparencies; clear aims and objectives; exercises; group activities; teaching sessions and aids; and support material and handouts.

£45   0-86242-254-X

If you would like to order any of these titles, please write to the address below, enclosing a cheque or money order for the appropriate amount made payable to Age Concern England. Credit card orders may be made on 020 8765 7200.

Mail Order Unit
Age Concern England
1268 London Road
London SW16 4ER

INFORMATION LINE

Age Concern produces over 40 comprehensive factsheets designed to answer many of the questions older people – or those advising them – may have, on topics such as:

- finding and paying for residential and nursing home care
- money benefits
- finding help at home
- legal affairs
- making a Will
- help with heating
- raising income from your home
- transfer of assets

Age Concern offers a factsheet subscription service that presents all the factsheets in a folder, together with regular updates throughout the year. The first year's subscription currently costs £65. Single copies (up to a maximum of five) are available free on receipt of an sae.

To order your FREE factsheet list, phone 0800 00 99 66 (a free call) or write to:

Age Concern
FREEPOST (SWB 30375)
Ashburton
Devon TQ13 7ZZ

LIST OF TABLES

Table	Page	Content
1	7	Food examples of the hierarchy of human need
2	15	Typical foods eaten by people from the Indian sub-continent, people of Chinese origin and people from the West Indies
3	20	Estimated average daily requirements for energy according to age and sex
4	24	Frequency of popular foods and drinks in the diets of older people
5	31	Percentage of older people with a specific nutrient deficiency according to blood analyses
6	33	Nutritional guidelines for community meals for older people
7	34	Sample menus for a community meal for an older person
8	36	Nutritional guidelines for food prepared for older people in residential and nursing homes
9	37	Sample menus for residential accommodation
10	45	Factors to consider in the service of meals
11	64	Sample meal plan for someone with diabetes
12	70	Dietary assessment techniques
13	82	Sample meal plan for offering snacks and enriching food
14	85	Factors that may result in a low fluid consumption
15	86	Sample list of drinks consumed in 24 hours by a carer
16	87	Sample food and fluid chart
17	91	Classification of modified thickness and textures – challenging and easier foods

INDEX